T

Our Journeys

Tubal Reversal

Our Journeys

by
Diana Dickherber

With special thanks to all of my TR sisters who were so generous to share their journeys!

Copyright © 2005
Diana Dickherber

All rights reserved. No part of this book may be reproduced in any form, except for the inclusion of brief quotations in a review, without permission in writing from the author or publisher.

Library of Congress Card Number: 2005908432

ISBN: 0-9773545-0-4

First Printing   October 2005

Additional copies of this book are available online at:

www.tubal-reversal-our-journeys-book.com

Printed in the U.S.A. by
Morris Publishing
3212 East Highway 30
Kearney, NE 68847
1-800-650-7888

This book is dedicated in memory of my father, Frank Michael Kowalczyk, Sr. Without him, and the Grace of God, this book would not have been possible.

And to all our unborn children yet to come:

For you created my inmost being; you knit me together in my mother's womb.

I praise you because I am fearfully and wonderfully made, I know that full well.

My frame was not hidden from you when I was made in the secret place.

When I was woven together in the depths of the earth, your eyes saw my unformed body.

All the days ordained for me were written in your book before one of them came to be.

Psalm 139:13-16

Contents

Introduction		ix.
Chapter 1	My Journey	1
Chapter 2	The Big Day Arrives	5
Chapter 3	Let Me Off This Ride	9
Chapter 4	Let Go, and Let God	11
Chapter 5	Melinda's Journey	21
Chapter 6	Jannette's Journey	25
Chapter 7	Heather's Journey	29
Chapter 8	Dawn's Journey	35
Chapter 9	Yvonne's Journey	39
Chapter 10	Amy's Journey	43
Chapter 11	Elaine's Journey	51
Chapter 12	Tori's Journey	55
Chapter 13	Denise's Journey	61

Chapter 14	Melissa's Journey	65
Chapter 15	Keri's Journey	67
Chapter 16	Christy's Journey	71
Chapter 17	Lori's Journey	75
Chapter 18	Bella's Journey	77
Chapter 19	Delores' Journey	83
Chapter 20	Kelli's Journey	89
Chapter 21	Laurie's Journey	97
Chapter 22	JoAnn's Journey	101
Chapter 23	Jennifer's Journey	109
Chapter 24	Maura's Journey	113
Chapter 25	Robin's Journey	119
Chapter 26	Liz's Journey	123
Chapter 27	Melanie's Journey	127
Chapter 28	Micaela's Journey	131
Chapter 29	Holly's Journey	135

Chapter 30 Quick Testimonies	139
Learn the Lingo	143
Angels Helping Others	147

Introduction

Let me begin by introducing myself. My name is Diana. I am a 32 year old stay at home, home-schooling mom with four beautiful blessings, one being a tubal reversal baby, who at the time of this writing is almost 2 ½ years old.

I wrote this book for several reasons. It's been in the making of my mind for quite some time. My primary reason for writing this book-not enough information on the subject. As a matter of fact, in my past four years of researching the subject of tubal reversals, I have come across nothing except information on the procedure itself. I wanted stories, true stories of those who have lived it first hand. I wanted to talk with women from all walks of life to find out where this journey has taken them from beginning to present. In presenting this book to you, I hope to bring alive what the journey is really like through the eyes of those who have lived it.

To those of you about to embark on this unknown, you are in for the ride of your life, possibly the most exciting adventure life may hold for you. I hope that through the journeys of myself and others, you will be more informed as you make that all important decision regarding a tubal reversal. I hope this book will bring you hope that having another child, a gift from God, can be not only a dream, but a reality.

To my TR sisters out there who have already had a reversal, wherever you are in your journey, may this book bless you and give you the courage and strength to ride out the storm. Finally, let us remember, whatever may be, it's in God's hands.

Diana Dickherber
Author

My Journey Begins
Chapter One

My journey to where I am now began back in the fall of 2001. We were new to the area, and were seeking out other families who did what we did, home-school. We met a family through our local support group, and they invited us to attend their church. Since we were seeking a new church family after our move anyway, we decided to give it a try. Little did I know that those few visits were about to set into motion a whole new thought pattern for me. A short while after joining the church, some new home-schooling friends of ours at the church were having difficulties with their pregnancy. Their unborn child was not well. To protect their privacy, I will not go into details, but will explain how this set God's plan for us into motion. One night, the church held a special meeting to pray over this family and their unborn child. The emotion in the room that evening, and the enormous faith of the parents as they poured their hearts out to God, was so amazing, and touched me in a way that was so intense, words could not describe it. That night, God showed me through these two friends, and their immense faith, just how precious life is. God had planted a new seed in my mind that was about to grow like wild fire.

As hard as this may be to believe, I woke the next morning, and informed my husband that I wanted to have a baby. I explained to him that I feel this is something God is telling us to do. He responded, "Okay, whatever you want to do." My husband, after nine years, knows that when I tell him God is speaking to me, big changes are coming soon. I've only heard God speaking to me loud and clear three times in my lifetime, this was one of them, and I knew it would be in my best interest to listen.

Immediately, I started researching everything I possibly could concerning tubal reversal. At this point, I didn't even know if it was possible. My mom had a friend who had the procedure successfully done back in the 1980's, but I assumed it was rarely a success. I came across several websites offering tubal reversal surgery, but one stood out among the rest, Dr. Gary Berger in Chapel Hill, North Carolina. I knew after reviewing his website and watching the amazing free video he sent to me on his procedure, regardless of the cost, this was my doctor of choice.

I let my husband Kevin know that I had made a decision on my doctor and was ready to get the ball rolling. He knows that when I put my mind to something, I want to take action immediately. I am not good at waiting. I just don't have much patience in that department. Although Dr. Berger's fees were very reasonable, it was still a lot of money to come up with on short notice. But I was determined that God would provide a way.

The next morning, I called Dr. Berger's office, and I proudly announced that I was ready to make an appointment. We paid the whole amount on three different credit cards, which looked silly, but again, I was determined. Luckily, my husband is a "wanted man" in his line of work, and we were able to pay the debt off very quickly.

I took the earliest appointment available that worked for us. That day, which I will never forget, was November 15, 2001. This gave me a whole month to obsess over this. It also gave me time to do more research and find others out there who have been through this procedure. I joined several online support groups which I found by typing tubal reversal into my groups search engine. I met a bunch of wonderful women on these groups, those who were saving for a reversal, those awaiting their big day like me, those on that rollercoaster ride we veterans call trying to conceive, and those who had already been blessed with one or more tubal reversal babies. I was full of questions. Regardless of how silly my questions may have seemed, several ladies were always willing to share their knowledge, and prepare me for that day, and the days to come. My online support groups were a Godsend. After four years, I still check in with some of the ladies from time to time, and probably always will. They saw me through my journey from the beginning until now, and were a wealth of information to me.

Psalm 40:1

I waited patiently for the Lord; he turned to me and heard my cry.

The Big Day Arrives
Chapter Two

The day I had been waiting for had finally arrived. I woke up on the morning before my surgery, packed and ready to go. One problem, I had a horrible sinus infection, high temperature, and felt awful. We headed out anyway, determined not to let anything hinder our plans. St. Louis, Missouri to Chapel Hill, North Carolina is quite a drive anyway, but driving while sick, I won't even go there. It was a very horrible experience.

We arrived at Dr. Berger's office for our consultation and an ultrasound that afternoon. From the minute I walked into the office, I knew I was in good hands and had made the right choice. I can only describe it as extreme peace, as though God was holding me in the palm of his hand, and he was.

After the ultrasound and some paperwork, it was over to meet Dr. Berger. It was wonderful to finally meet the man that I had heard so much about. Dr. Berger was the first doctor I had met that wasn't anxious to run us out the door and move on to his next patient. He took plenty of time out of his busy schedule to get to know us, ask us some general questions, and just helping us to make sure this was what we really wanted.

The anesthesiologist was our next stop. She filled me in on what to expect on the big day. Of course, she noticed that horrible cold I had, and showed enough concern to suggest putting the surgery off. I was crushed, but tried to understand. I explained that it took us over fourteen hours to drive here, and it would be a long time before I would be able to reschedule. I was informed to go to the hotel and rest, take some medication, and arrive as scheduled for surgery. If all was okay, the surgery would be a go. If not, I would have no choice but to reschedule. Needless to say, I was determined that my surgery would take place as planned. I performed some serious doctoring on myself, and got some much needed rest.

We arrived at the stated time the next morning. I prayed the whole way over that everything would work out okay. I still felt horrible, but prayed for a miracle. The anesthesiologist looked me over, took my temperature and vitals, and gave me the okay. I was ecstatic to say the least! At first, I was devastated thinking that the surgery may have had to been put on hold, but looking back now, I really appreciate the fact that the staff cared enough about me to postpone the surgery, if it meant going forward with it could be harmful to me in any way.

I was taken back to get prepped, which was basically the same as if you were going into any other surgery. That was the last thing I remembered. I woke up in the operating room at one point. I asked one of the attending nurses if everything was okay. She responded with, "Dr. Berger has some great news for you." That's all I needed to know. I dozed back off for a short time, and woke again in the recovery room. I was quick to "snap out" of it, so to speak. I asked when I could speak to Dr. Berger. I also asked when I could leave. I felt great and wanted to go. Dr. Berger came by a short time later and gave me the wonderful news. He said everything looked great. I was left with 9 cm of tube on each side. For those of you who aren't familiar with normal tube lengths, this was considered excellent. I have read that normal tube length at birth is 9-10 cm on average. Dr. Berger stated to me that whoever performed my tubal ligation was very kind to me.

The next morning, one of the nurses came to visit us at the hotel room. I was told what to expect during my recovery, given some medications, and told what to do and what not to do. We headed back home that morning very excited.

I look back on my recovery and realize it was a breeze. I did not need any of the pain medication prescribed to me, and I was up and back to just about normal in a couple days. My incision healed quickly, and I was for the most part pain free through the whole recovery.

I knew that regardless of the outcome, I felt whole again. I had reversed the mistake I had chosen to make six years ago, and have never looked back or had any regrets.

Psalm 130:5

I wait for the Lord, my soul waits, and in his word I put my hope.

Let Me Off This Ride!
Chapter 3

The reversal procedure was complete, and I was officially on my way! I had hopped aboard the rollercoaster ride us veterans call TTC (trying to conceive). I didn't know it at the time, but this would soon become the bumpiest part of my journey yet. Our faith was about to be put to the test in a big way.

I will fess up now before I even begin. I am not proud about some of the information that I plan to share with you. But I believe it is best to be upfront and honest about what kind of effect trying to conceive a baby post tubal reversal can have on a person. I think it best to inform you ahead of time, so you may have an idea of what to expect. Hopefully, by learning from my mistakes, what I put myself, my husband, and my children through, will never apply to you.

We tried to conceive right away in November. By Christmas, I was already wondering why I wasn't pregnant. I had this idea in my head that since I read all the fertility books on charting my cycle, had great tube lengths, and was taking this concoction and that, that I would immediately become pregnant. I couldn't have been more wrong. As my OBGYN once put it, just because the tubes are now "fixed" does not make them "functional". I was hoping I would not fall into that category.

I survived the first month of bad news. I figured anyhow that in the next month or two I would get that big positive. But the next couple months came and passed, as well as some more after that, and still no pregnancy. By this point, I had already become an emotional wreck. Trying to conceive a child soon became a chore, and negative after negative HPT (home pregnancy test) brought my spirits down even further. I wore myself out with monitoring my temperature at the same time every morning, along with trying to keep track of other signs to indicate ovulation was approaching. As much as I hate to admit it, let the truth be told, I believe my husband was beginning to feel like nothing more than a sperm donor. I don't mean to offend with that, but I must tell it like it was. My poor children were not getting the time with me that they needed either. I home schooled all three children at the time, and I wasn't exactly the best teacher during all of this. I was too caught up in myself at the time to focus on anything else for long. I had all but given up at this point. Something had to give.

Let Go, and Let God
Chapter 4

It was early June, and the frustration of no pregnancy had finally gotten the best of me. I remember this day as clearly as if it were yesterday. I was devastated and felt their was no longer any hope. To make matters worse, I knew I wasn't putting my faith in God the way I should. After seven short months, I had hit rock bottom with this. I called out to God in prayer and asked him to take this desire to have a child away from me, and let me leave my fertility issues in His hands, which is where they belonged anyway. I had given this prayer to God before, but this time I immediately felt at peace, and this time I left it with God, for good. I asked God to speak to me about what he wanted from me, what did he have for me if this wasn't it. I knew I was put here on this earth for a reason, I just didn't know what that reason was yet. I was soon to find out.

As I had stated earlier, I have only heard God speaking to me loud and clear a few times in my life. Once, when he called me to home-educate the children, and secondly, when he placed it upon my heart to get that reversal. Little did I know at the time, but the Lord was about to put both myself, and my husband, Kevin, to the biggest test of faith we had ever seen, and may ever see again.

I am a firm believer that when in doubt it's God's voice you hear, look for confirmation from other sources. For days, I had this feeling inside me that something wasn't quite right, but I couldn't put my finger on it. Little did I know, Kevin was getting these same feelings, at the same time I was. We were the confirmation for each other, as you will soon see. Now bear with me here. I am sure you are wondering by now what this has to do with trying to conceive, but you will see, this was all a part of God's great plan to get us to that point.

Kevin and I talked that evening about the day's events, as usual. Somehow or another, the topic of these odd feelings came up in the conversation. To cut to the chase, we had decided that night that God was telling us to sell everything and move to Tennessee. We learned soon that God wanted us to go, but not to Tennessee. We had the right idea, go, but we were only partly listening to God's will for us. We added our own desires into His plan, too.

With the go ahead from God, we did what most would call the absolutely unthinkable. Although family and friends didn't make any negative comments toward us, we know deep down that they must have thought we went off the deep end, and should be committed. We told the kids we were packing up our 19 ft. travel trailer and heading out on the mission field, starting with Oregon. That's right, Oregon. It didn't take us long to figure out that when God said go, he had a plan for when we got there. A church in Oregon needed help completing their new building, and God was sending us on our way with nothing but one plastic tote a piece for personal belongings, meaning clothes, mainly. We had a huge yard sale and sold everything, absolutely everything that we owned. What took us six years together to accumulate, was gone in a weekend. We rented our home to our pastor, and left July 5, 2002, for Phoenix, Oregon. We said goodbye to friends, family, and even our pets, and headed down our own Oregon Trail.

I would love to share all of our wonderful memories of that trip, but that would be another book in itself. We did spend three months in Oregon, and it was the best time of our life. Kevin spent his time building the church. I spent mine helping at summer camp and teaching VBS and a Wednesday night children's class. We had never been more at peace, had more time together, and bonded as a family the way we did during our time in Oregon. We lived day to day and depended on God to meet all of our needs, but the stress of the everyday bump and grind was completely non-existent. I believe this may have contributed to our success in becoming pregnant during that trip.

I am one of those women who just knows when I am pregnant. I can just sense it. About the second week of August, even before old Aunt Flo (menstruation) was due, I had that feeling. I have never been one to have morning sickness, or any complications whatsoever, so I rely on my gut instinct. I was pretty hesitant to take an HPT yet, because I did not want to get caught up in that vicious cycle once again. On September 13, 2002, I purchased an HPT. At 4:00 a.m., the next morning, I discovered I was pregnant. Now don't laugh, but as many women do, I had brilliant ideas in my head of how I would tell Kevin the good news that he would soon be a dad again. I thought I'd mail him a card, or buy a cute baby gift, etc, etc, etc. But, like a woman gone mad, I run into our room and present him with a used HPT. What a rude awakening! I said, "Do you know what this means?" He said, "Yeah, it means you might be pregnant." I replied, "No, it means I am." I'm sure I don't need to tell you, but I couldn't go back to sleep.

The next day, I immediately contacted Dr. Berger's office and an OBGYN as instructed by Dr. Berger himself. I knew exactly what tests I needed done, and I knew what information I was to share with them. Our insurance was useless in Oregon, but I found a midwife at the health department in Medford. I let her know that I had a tubal reversal, the date of my LMP (last menstrual period), and that I was at an increased risk for an ectopic pregnancy. She drew the necessary blood work and examined me. She asked if my dates were correct because from what she gathered from the examination, I was either carrying twins or was further along than what I thought. She sent me to the hospital for an ultrasound. I was only five weeks into my pregnancy, so when they saw only a sac, they were not concerned. I was told to relax, the baby was in the right place, and not in the tube. I was thrilled! I called everyone right away to tell the good news. I praised God, knowing that we were being blessed with this baby because of our obedience to him, meaning carrying out the will he had for us. We would soon learn, that although God will call us to go, that doesn't mean he will have us stay. I think sometimes God's just checking to see if we will act in faith.

I got a call from the midwife a week later. She wanted me to go back to the hospital for another ultrasound. I was happy because I knew we would see a heartbeat by now. Everything I have read states a heartbeat would be seen by 5-6 weeks. At this time, I was slightly past six weeks. I was brought into the ultrasound room and excitedly waited to see the heartbeat. We never saw it. It is not customary for the technician to give results, but she did. She stated to me that we should have seen more than a sac by now. Diagnosis, blighted ovum. This baby was not a keeper.

I went to see the midwife before heading back to the trailer. I just couldn't face Kevin and the kids at that moment. I told her the technician diagnosed the pregnancy a blighted ovum and asked her what I should do. She told me I should see an OBGYN here locally. I let her know that I would be heading home to see my own. I was then encouraged to see an OBGYN for a D&C before leaving town. I was informed of the dangers of miscarriage and was advised against taking the chance driving home through the desert in case I were to miscarry and not be able to reach help. She was worried that I might hemorrhage. I had already made up my mind to head home to resolve this, and was I ever glad I did.

I headed back to the trailer, knowing I had to get this over with. I was in tears the rest of the day, and for the first time in my life I was angry with God. Why would he bring us this far, only to take our child away from us? Haven't we been obedient? Haven't we stepped out on faith, all the way? I know my husband did the best he could to comfort and reassure me, but he just didn't understand.

My anger towards God was very short lived. Remember the family I told you about in the beginning, the one with the unborn child that was having complications. Something my friend's husband had once told me came to my mind that day, and will always be one of the wisest pieces of advice I have, or will ever receive. He had once told me to praise God in all situations. Let me say it again, because it holds a lot of truths, "Praise God in all situations." That day, the meaning of that message hit me all at once. We should not only praise God in the good, but also in the times when life hits a bump. We should praise God in our trials, too, because as always, God sees the bigger picture, and He sometimes uses those trials for His own good purposes. They help us to grow!

The day before we left for home, we got some bad news from my husband's sister. There were some complications with the rental situation that needed immediate attention. We began to wonder if God didn't use this pregnancy loss to get us home. Like I said before, he asked us to go, but that didn't mean he would keep us there. We thought maybe God wanted to see if we would even go to begin with.

I left Oregon in good spirits. I praised God, as crazy as it may sound to some, for the loss of this baby. I knew God had a plan and His reasons. I had an appointment to see my OBGYN on October 8, 2002, to discuss the option of a D&C.

I walked into the office of my OBGYN that morning ready to discuss the options. I was hoping the baby would have passed on it's own by then, but it didn't. My body still thought it was pregnant, eight weeks by then. My doctor came in, and I explained the whole situation to him. He asked if it was okay for him to do an ultrasound. I told him of course, although I didn't see the point in it. There would be nothing to see but an empty sac. I reasoned that the ultrasound was routine before doing a D&C, so nothing further was discussed. I was taken to the ultrasound room, which was heartbreaking. That day, several women before me were probably overjoyed at the view of the beating heart of their unborn little ones, and oohing and ahhing over little body parts. It was about more than I could bear.

As I sat there waiting, I thought about all the miracles Jesus performed when he walked this earth. I was reminded, miracles didn't happen only then, they happen today, too. I immediately prayed to God, without really expecting a response, letting him know that I am aware of His ability to work a miracle. I acknowledged the fact that if He wanted this baby to be alive and well, then he had the power to do it. Although I wholeheartedly believed that, I didn't expect a miracle to take place that day.

I lay back on the table, forgetting about my recent prayer, and let my doctor proceed with the ultrasound. I watched with hope, looking to see that empty sac one more time, but what I saw was a sac with a rapidly blinking dot, the heart of my precious baby. She was alive and well. I am in tears as I relive this moment right now because it was truly a day of joy! God had worked a miracle that day! I truly believe that while in Oregon, God had hidden my unborn child from our view to see how we would respond to thinking our child was not a keeper. As I stated earlier, I was angry with God, but for a very short time, before I was down on my knees seeking forgiveness. Had I stayed angry with God, we may not have had our child today. I firmly believe that our leaping out on faith and acting in obedience to God, is the only reason we have her today. I know that God rewards our obedience, and he showers us with wonderful gifts, although we deserve none of them.

My pregnancy was pretty uneventful. I did worry quite a bit about the well-being of the baby, though. Although nothing was ever wrong with her, I had that mindset that there was at one time, and that I needed to be extra cautious.

Right around the time of my due date, my doctor and I discussed the delivery and what to expect, although I pretty much had that figured out by now. He assumed I would be having an epidural. I corrected him by saying, "No remember, I am having her natural, with nothing." He told me I was crazy.

Why would I want to go through that pain? We both laughed! On a medical level, I suppose he was right, but what he didn't understand was that I felt it was something I had to do. This baby was a miracle, and I wanted to make sure I didn't miss a thing. I didn't want any regrets, later wishing I had done things differently.

I had my mind made up about a name for a girl almost immediately. My gut instinct told me she was a girl from the beginning. I knew this was not an ordinary baby, as no reversal baby is. They are miracles, precious gifts from God, as all children are. He did not have to bless us with this child. I knew no ordinary name was going to do. I wanted every part of her name to be biblical, my way of glorifying God, was through her name.

On May 13th, 2003, at 10:48 a.m., Hannah Elizabeth Grace was brought into this earth by the Grace of God! I will never forget that day, or the joy of seeing her beautiful little face for the first time. The baby that I had hoped and dreamed for was here, and she was our little blessing, our little piece of heaven.

One piece of advice I would give to others seeking a reversal is to go for it. If it is God's will, you will have that baby. If not, at least you acted in obedience to his word, turning your fertility back over to Him, into the hands of our Creator, where it belongs.

Psalm 46:10

Be still, and know that I am God…

Melinda's Journey
Chapter 5

I met Melinda online through the testimonial pages on Dr. Berger's website. Melinda is 34 years old. She had her reversal on November 5, 2001, just days before mine. But unlike my story, Melinda became pregnant immediately. Here is Melinda's story.

My name is Melinda. I was 34 years old when I found the wonderful Dr. Berger. I had my tubes tied in 1992, and divorced a few years later. I was saddened when I heard the news in my area of the high cost, time needed off work, and low success rates of having your tubes reconnected. I had remarried, and my husband was an only child. He was a great dad to my then 6 year old son, but also desired to be a father to biological children of his own.

One day through desperation, I felt the presence of God. I typed in reversal on my search engine and found a link to the website for Dr. Berger. I began reading the testimonials and cried over many. I decided to print them out to read again. I read the website from front to finish many times as well. Skeptical, yet excited, I talked it over with my husband and our son, and all were happy. They encouraged me and supported us in our decision to have the reversal in hopes for another child.

My surgery was November 5, 2001. I was able to conceive on December 10th of the same year. I had a positive urine and blood test on December 20, 2001. My husband Bob did not believe I was pregnant after the 4:00 a.m. urine test. That is why we had the blood test as well. My family physician was really skeptical as well. When he walked into the room with the results, he was smiling from ear to ear. He gave me the biggest hug and a congratulations, mama. Bob was amazed we were pregnant just one short month after surgery. What a glorious Christmas present we had for everyone!

Below is the poem my husband wrote in only four days to give to his grandmother. He is very close to her. She was so worried we would get our hopes up, only to have them crushed. We were truly blessed by God, and we owe it all to the Lord and Saviour.

A Christmas Riddle

There once was a boy, with hair shiny red;
He fell in love with a girl, and soon they were wed.
They bought themselves a house, made of brick, not log;
For a pet they had a cat, then they bought themselves a dog.
They both had to work, so the bills would get paid;
Her job was in town at *** hearing aid.
His job was to travel, to deliver uniforms and a mat.
But as time continued on, they both began to get fat.
"A diet we shall start," is what they both did claim;
But the expert said, "No way!" your reasons are not the same.

To the boy, he said, "You eat too much!"
"Cut back today, or you'll have to skip lunch."
To the girl, he said, "A totally different reason."
What a perfect time for good news, in this joyous season.
Now that this riddle, has gone along way to far;
If you still need help to solve it, just wish upon a star.
For this CHRISTmas surprise, indeed, is not just a mishap;
Now for the 13th time, you're going to become,
Great-GrandNan and Great-GrandPap.

Jenna Shay was born August 16, 2002. We were even more blessed six months later when we conceived again and gave birth to another beautiful girl on December 1, 2003. We named her Becca Rene.

Today, they are almost two and three. I enjoy every moment, yet will not deny that this has been harder than I ever thought. I have been blessed with a ton of support from family, friends, Dr. Berger, and his staff. Dr. Berger's staff were a great support during the ups and downs I had while waiting for the HCG test and ultrasounds to come back normal. At one time, Patty from Dr. Berger's office said I should be a poster child for them, referring to the fact that I conceived so quickly both pregnancies.

I was even lucky enough to see Jenna's picture on the newly designed web site of Dr. Berger with my e-mail attached. I have had the honor of talking with many women who have had the surgery, or were contemplating whether or not to. I thank God and Dr. Berger every day for my beautiful girls. Yes, even on those trying days when I am dead tired, and they seem to pull every toy out they can and do all the wrong things. Like now, I cannot see my floor, but the beautiful sound of voices playing fill the air, and make it all better.

Jannette's Journey
Chapter 6

Jannette's story really touched my heart. After having her dreams come crashing down, she did not give up. This story is like so many others, the word reversal suddenly pops into our vocabulary, and we become women on a mission. Here is Jannette's story.

My name is Jannette Wasserman. This is a story about the miracles that happened in my life due to a procedure called tubal reversal. I had two children from a previous marriage. I was remarried in 1999 to a wonderful man, my husband, Perri. We both love each other very much and just accepted the fact that we couldn't have children together due to a tubal ligation.

One day, I was reading a magazine, and came across an article about tubal reversal surgery. After reading that article, I began research, and became obsessed with having the procedure done myself. I typed tubal reversal in a search engine. Many sites came up. But the one that interested me the most was Dr. Gary Berger's website. I read the whole thing, called to order the free video, and watched it. I then showed the tape to my husband, Perri, and he agreed we should go for it. I called Dr. Berger's office to ask where to begin. I was told to get a copy of my post-operative report from my tubal ligation. I was very happy with what I read. I had hulka clips, one of the easiest ligations to successfully reverse. I faxed the post-operative report to Dr Berger's office. Shortly after, I received a call from his office stating I was a prime candidate for surgery.

I live in Pennsylvania, and wondered how we would get to Chapel Hill. My husband, after finding out where it was, realized his fraternity brother lived within two miles of Dr. Berger's office. As fate would have it, I had my reversal and was amazed to have no pain, just some slight discomfort. After the surgery, we started trying right away and were pregnant three months later. Words cannot explain the feeling you have when you find yourself to be pregnant for the first time post reversal. I am crying now as I think of that day. To be able to give the man I love so very much a child: Priceless!

Little did I know, this pregnancy would come to an end. I began working at a pediatrician's office about a month into my pregnancy. I had contracted Fifth's disease, which is similar to chicken pox. In the early stages of pregnancy it can cause a stillbirth. During my four month checkup, the doctor could no longer detect a heartbeat. I was sent to the hospital for an ultrasound. No one said anything, but I knew there was nothing. They would have showed me a healthy heartbeat on the screen if there had been one. I had to return to my midwife to hear what I already knew. I got sick. I couldn't believe this. Everything was happening so fast. It just didn't seem true. I was in complete shock.

I was too far into the pregnancy for a D&C. I was given a drug to induce labor. Six and a half hours later, I gave birth to my baby boy, Jax Lane Wassermann. The baby boy I had dreamed of was gone. I was able to hold my little boy and see every detail of his little body. I still have his picture, which at first I thought was a morbid idea, but taken from a distance it was done very tastefully. I even have his little footprints. I think it is very important to have had all these things to help put some closure on our tragedy.

Time off work was horrible for me. It's funny how you don't realize the effect something such as this has on a person until it happens to you. I couldn't believe all the women I knew that had miscarriages and never said anything before, or how common miscarriage is.

Going back to work was worse than the time off. Again, I worked in a pediatrician's office, and it was heartbreaking to see all the newborns on a daily basis when I didn't have mine. I must have cried daily for months. I decided that was it. I was on a mission. I needed to be pregnant right away. Two months later it happened, I was pregnant. I was just as happy and excited as the first time. As time went on I had to quit my job. I became paranoid of every sick child that came into the office. I wasn't willing to give another baby up due to a child coming in with an illness that could harm my baby.

Everything with this pregnancy went well. I gave birth to a healthy 8lb., 6oz. red-haired little girl. She was the most beautiful thing in the world. I enjoyed every moment with her, even waking several times a night to feed her. I actually looked forward to it. She was pure joy! All I could think of was having another child right away. I believe all children should have at least one sibling to grow up with. Six months later, I was pregnant again and ecstatic to say the least. Nine months later, on September 13, 2003, I gave birth to another baby girl. She was 8lbs., 5 ½ oz. My girls are my pride and joy. They do something adorable everyday, several times a day. I am amazed at how beautiful and smart they are. They are so much like my husband and I. One looks like him, one looks like me.

My little boy Jax will never be forgotten. He is buried with my father and my little brother all in one grave. I know they are taking care of him as I would have. I now have three angels looking over my girls. I thank God every day for the miracles he blessed us with. I look forward to every stage in their lives, and enjoy every day that I spend with them. I also have to thank Dr. Berger. I am so grateful for what he has helped do in our lives. He is truly a great doctor and man.

Heather's Journey
Chapter 7

Heather's story is very similar to mine. We both needed the experience of another's tragedy to wake us up to what really counts in life. I think we all need to take the message in her journey and begin to live. We cannot number our own days on this earth, only the Lord can, and you need take each one of them and "live like you were dying."

My name is Heather. I have been married to my husband, Mark, for 18 years now. We have three daughters, Jessica, 18, Caitlin, 16, and Taylor, 14. We also have our tubal reversal miracles, Jake, who is 4, and Joey, who will be 2 shortly. Yes, that makes five, and we are incredibly blessed. I am about to turn 41 and my husband 43. The boys will keep us young I hope.

I suppose our story begins 18 years ago. All I really wanted to do at that point was to be a mom. I became pregnant with Jessica in the dating phase of our relationship. Although not planned, she was very much wanted from day one. She came into our home at the perfect time and brought such joy and laughter into the house. How could we not do this baby thing again? Caitlin was born 23 months later, followed by Taylor, 2 ½ years after that. Life was busy, never enough money, but always an abundance of love. I had a few issues in all of my pregnancies. At the urging of my OBGYN, I had a tubal ligation at the time of my last C-section. Sounded alright at the time. I just wanted to deliver a healthy baby, and I did not give a lot of thought about how I would feel after.

I signed those waiver papers practically on the delivery table. It was literally the next day that I wondered what I had done. My regret was instant and my sadness immeasurable. My husband was understanding, but let's face it, when you are the sole breadwinner of the family the daunting task of providing is enormous. He supported me emotionally the best he could, but could never truly understand where I was coming from.

Life went on. Babies of friends and family were born. With each birth, I would become so sad and ache for another baby to hold and nurse. I struggled with the greed factor, too. How selfish was I to want another baby, when some have never experienced the joy once. Or what about those who have given birth and lost a baby, a toddler, or a teen. Who was I to think I should have another baby in my life?

Each year, Mark and I would go away for our anniversary, and each year we would spend a portion of our time talking about my desire to have a baby in our lives. It became ritual conversation, one I believe he came to dread. Not because he didn't love me, but because he felt complete. He yearned to make me happy, but felt he had given all he had to give. I didn't resent him, I understood, but nonetheless, I was always left with that pit in my stomach.

In the year 2000, we headed out on our yearly journey. During a stop for lunch, he began the conversation by saying, "Let's just get the talk over now instead of later in the weekend." My heart sank, but instead of disappointment, I could not believe what I heard. He said, "Let's do it." I was dumbfounded. I asked him what set about a change of heart after 10 years. He said that all these years he truly prayed for God to guide him, to one day give him the peace in his own mind that his decision of three children were enough. But God's answer was for Mark to open his heart to the possibility of more.

An important part of our journey is what happened the following year. We lost a family friend to Leukemia. That process was so incredibly sad, but so filled with blessings at the same time. We watched this family lose their mother. I was there the day she took her last breath. I was part of such a personal, heart-breaking journey of someone's life. We walked away seeing the true meaning of being here on this earth. Living, loving each other, helping our fellow man when God calls you, is what really matters. House payments, car payments, college, etc., will work itself out. Live today and love each other today. I give the credit of my boys' lives to my friend, Pat, and her family. If not for their courage, the true meaning of life may not have become so clear to me.

I went home that very weekend and got on the computer to search for information on tubal reversals. God lead me to Dr. Berger's website. I was sure this was it. I made the phone calls, made all the appointments and reservations, and in three short weeks, I was on a plane with my best friend to Chapel Hill. We didn't tell anyone about this. Mark stayed home with the girls. We told everyone else that my friend and I were on our way to a spa in Arizona. I arrived in Chapel Hill on a Monday, had my consult on Tuesday, surgery on Wednesday, and home to California on Thursday, as simple, and as complicated as that.

We decided, what ever was meant to be, would be, which is the advice I would give to anyone. If you are a person of faith, put that faith in God and let Him guide you. Follow your dreams, follow your heart, and be patient. It is in His time.

I was one of the lucky ones. I left the operating room with tube lengths of 7 cm and 6.5 cm. I was 36 years old, in good health, and in good shape. The very next month we were pregnant. Jake Matthew arrived the following spring. We decided if we got pregnant again, great, if not, we wouldn't be disappointed. Well, lo and behold, I became pregnant again, and Joseph arrived September 2003. I am so lucky they have each other since there is such an age difference between our girls and our boys.

Our lives are enriched for the mere fact of their being. They bring such joy to our lives. Their sisters adore them, and they their sisters. I cannot imagine our lives without them. Dr. Berger will never be forgotten in the Needham household. He truly gave us a second chance at the gift of life. I once said that not a day in my life will go by that I won't look in the eyes of my sons and thank God for giving us a doctor such as Dr. Berger. Our simple thanks will never suffice. A thank you seems so trivial, but he hasn't even asked for that. He is a humble man.

Luke 1:45

Blessed is she who has believed that what the Lord has said to her will be accomplished!

Dawn's Journey
Chapter 8

I am sure you will find Dawn's story very unusual and quite unique! I have met couples seeking a tubal reversal. I have met couples wanting to reverse a vasectomy. But never have I met a couple within the same marriage who had done both. Here is Dawn's story.

After the birth of our third child, my husband had a vasectomy. After three kids, in three years, we felt we could not afford anymore. I always kept that feeling that I wanted more. In 1995, we starting looking into having a vasectomy reversal. We were told that having it reversed was not covered by our insurance, so we began putting money aside, saving to have the procedure done. Later, we found out that the insurance we had would cover the reversal as long as they did not pay for the vasectomy to begin with. So in August, my husband had the vasectomy reversal, paying only a $100.00 co-pay. I found out in June that I was pregnant. My son was born in 1997, with four more siblings following close behind.

Eight children later, I had my tubes tied in February 2002. I regretted it the day I had it done. I felt like I made the decision for everyone else. After all, isn't eight kids enough. That's what everyone kept saying.

In January 2003, we started talking about having a tubal reversal. My OBGYN referred us to a local hospital. We were told it would cost around $20,000, with not much experience from the doctor. I left the hospital with very little hope. That summer, I searched the internet for more options. I found Dr. Berger. Everything I researched on the internet lead me back to him. My husband was very skeptical, but agreed to give it a shot.

In September 2003, I called and scheduled my surgery for November 10th. I mailed them a bank check overnight and started making arrangements. Everything fell into place and time flew very quickly. I knew from the moment I called Chapel Hill, I had made the right decision. I was never nervous, and my surgery went as scheduled.

I had my first period on November 17, 2003, and found out that I was pregnant on December 10, 2003. I was pregnant exactly one month after surgery. I delivered a very happy and healthy baby boy on July 29, 2004. We knew we wanted one more. In February 2005, we found out we were expecting our second reversal baby. Our due date this time is November 10, 2005, two years from the anniversary of my tubal reversal. This time we are expecting a girl. My husband is so excited. She will probably make her appearance mid-October. All of my children have been 3-5 weeks early.

There is not a day that goes by that I don't thank God for leading me to Dr. Berger and all of his wonderful staff at Chapel Hill. Without Him, we would not have our miracle and a second one on the way. Ten children later, we have decided to stop for now, but who knows what the future will bring.

Genesis 1:28a

God blessed them and said, "Be fruitful and increase in number; fill the earth and subdue it"

Yvonne's Journey
Chapter 9

I found Yvonne's story interesting because her husband initiated the idea for Yvonne to get a tubal reversal. I find the opposite to be true in most cases, and find a story such as theirs refreshing. Here is Yvonne's story.

My name is Yvonne Hyde. Dr. Berger performed my reversal in October 2001, and I delivered via C-section, Alysan Paige Hyde, on December 20, 2002.

I had my tubes tied after my two sons were born, Mitch in 1990 and Bryan in 1993. Mitch was a preemie born at 33 weeks and weighing a mere 4 lbs., 13 oz. We had a few touchy weeks with him, but all turned out well. Two years later, Bryan was born three weeks early. I had toxemia during both pregnancies and had to endure a lot of bed rest. I had decided no more. I had my tubes tied at the end of 1993. Unfortunately, I was a divorced mom three years later.

I thought it would always just be the boys and I. But in October 1998, I met Gerald. We were married in July 1999. Gerald had a daughter, Heather, from a previous marriage. Our families blended very well and we were all doing great. Absolutely out of the blue one day, I received a dozen beautiful red roses at work. A day or so later, my husband popped the idea of a baby on me. I was very unsure at first.

I felt a little too old at 33 and was scared of starting over. I was afraid that since my pregnancies weren't exactly smooth when I was younger, that surely they would hold more complications now.

I agreed though and began researching doctors right away. Fortunately, we live only about an hour from Chapel Hill, so I found Dr. Berger almost immediately. He had the best success rate I could find. I scheduled right away before I lost my nerve.

The week of the procedure, I was so nervous. I had two previous C-sections which made me hesitant to have another abdominal surgery. But the staff was absolutely wonderful and made me feel at ease from the start. Before I knew it, I was in the recovery room surprisingly pain free. I felt so well, that instead of staying overnight, we went directly home. I must admit, I felt so good, I didn't exactly follow the rest and no driving rules. I had the procedure on a Thursday and was back to work by Monday.

I really didn't expect to get pregnant right away, if at all, but I did. We were so excited! My OBGYN considered me at risk due to previous toxemia and premature delivery. We both kept waiting for something to go wrong, but it didn't. I never suffered from morning sickness, high blood pressure, excess weight, etc. I did not have any complications at all. I guess she was just meant to be.

On December 20th, I had a scheduled C-section at 8:00 a.m. Paige was born a happy, healthy 7 lb.

baby. I felt so great after the birth, I was released the next morning. I came home with her in time to have the best Christmas I'd had in a long time.

Paige will be three this year. When I look at her it's still hard to believe sometimes that she is here and she's mine. She is a constant joy and has been a great baby. I have had many women write to me from Dr. Berger's website. I encourage everyone who writes to have that reversal. It works!

Psalm 30:11,12

You turned my wailing into dancing; you removed my sackcloth and clothed me with joy, that my heart may sing to you and not be silent. O Lord my God, I will give you thanks forever.

Amy's Journey
Chapter 10

Amy really encouraged me to never give up. She stayed strong and determined from beginning to end, and the end result was priceless. Amy is proof that dreams really do come true! Here is Amy's story!

My name is Amy. I am currently 31 years old with three children, one of which I had after my tubal reversal surgery. I was married to a man for about eight years. Three of those years were good years. We had our first daughter our first year of marriage, and had our second daughter our third year of marriage. It was an abusive relationship and I was not happy. I felt I didn't need to bring more children into a bad situation, so I decided to have a tubal ligation. I had a bilateral cauterization when I was 26 years old. My marriage ended a few years later.

I actually met my current husband in high school. We had dated briefly after high school, but decided to end our relationship on good terms and go our separate ways. But here we are again years later, still very much in love with each other. This time we wanted to try to make it work. He had never been married and had no children. He has loved my children as his own from the moment we got back together, but we knew we would have to think about our relationship and what not being able to have biological children of his own would mean to him. I had to know if I couldn't give him a child of his own, that he would still want to continue a relationship with me. This was a discussion we had many times during the first year we were dating. He decided he would love me, with or without a child of his own, and proposed to me on Thanksgiving Day in front of all of our family. With tears in my eyes, I accepted.

The realization of spending the rest of my life with this man and not having a child with him hit me very hard one day. I began to research the procedure to have my tubal ligation reversed, if even possible. I read books, and I spent many hours on the internet researching anything and everything I could regarding the tubal reversal procedure. I called doctors, nurses, and women who had already had a reversal. I spent hours on message boards soaking up information like a sponge. No matter where I went, or who I talked to, one name kept resurfacing above the others, Dr. Gary Berger.

I then became a woman on a mission. I researched Dr. Berger. I compared his education and post surgery statistics against other doctors who perform the same surgery, and I chatted online with several of his patients. All of the information I was gathering seemed "too good to be true." Could there actually be a procedure out there performed by a skilled doctor that might actually allow me to have a child with the man I love? The answer was a resounding, "yes!"

It made me nervous to consider having a reversal done so far from our home in Arkansas, but we began to call Chapel Hill to find out more information from the staff there. How long would I be off work? Could my husband stay with me in the recovery room after surgery? How was it possible to do this on an outpatient basis? What about after I came home? And the final most important question, how much does the procedure cost? The staff at Chapel Hill were able to answer all of my questions without hesitation and to my complete satisfaction. The cost of the procedure was something we would have to work on. In the meantime, the staff offered to send us the free videotape of the procedure itself, so we could watch it and decide for ourselves.

We spent many nights watching that video over and over. So encouraged that there were others out there that had a reversal done and were having children again. We decided to go with Dr. Berger and his staff at Chapel Hill. It was the right decision for us.

We started saving our money for our procedure costs and our trip to North Carolina. We were so excited about the chance to have a child together. We created a chart of sorts that looked like a baby bottle. It had increments of dollar amounts on the side to keep track of how much we had saved and how much we still needed to save to have the reversal done. We'd mark off a little bit more each week. The baby bottle was filling ever so slowly. We were excited, but began to grow very impatient.

Without my knowledge, my husband began to take matters into his own hands. He came home one day with a big bouquet of flowers in a ceramic baby carriage with two baby rattles attached. His hands were shaking as he handed me the flowers and asked me to read the card inside. The card said, "The time has come for us to fulfill our dreams." I had no idea what the card meant, or what he was trying to tell me. Then he smiled real big and told me we had gotten approved for a loan, and we were going to be able to get the surgery done sooner than we had ever dreamed! We called Chapel Hill and scheduled the reversal at the earliest date possible. We made arrangements for the older girls to stay home, so they could continue to go to school. On February 9, 2004, we were off to Chapel Hill, North Carolina to pursue our dreams.

The visit with the staff the day before the procedure was anything but typical. I expected a strict, uptight surgical environment with stiff, stern nurses. What I saw was completely opposite. The office was very cozy and inviting. The staff was warm and welcoming. Even Dr. Berger was very friendly. He took the time to sit with us and talk one on one about the decision we had made. I knew from this moment on, this was the best decision we could have made. I knew we would have no regrets about choosing this facility and Dr. Berger.

We returned to our hotel room that afternoon. Neither one of us could sleep well that night. We got up bright and early the next morning, anxious to get to the clinic. Once again, the OR nurses were just as friendly as the office staff, making sure I was comfortable and calm. They were sure to see that I knew what was going on and exactly what would happen, step by step. I felt very at ease with the whole process. Before I knew it, I was off to sleep so Dr. Berger could do his work.

I woke up to the sight of my husband by my side and a nurse speaking softly to me. As soon as the nurse knew I was aware enough to comprehend anything, she began to explain to me how the procedure went and began to encourage me to begin my recovery process. I was left with 5 cm of tube on my right side and 4.5 cm of tube on my left side. Both sides appeared to be open and good.

Once back at the hotel, I was very at ease the rest of the day. I dozed on and off. My husband never left my side. The next morning, a nurse from the clinic came to my hotel room to check on me and look over my incision. She gave me a good report, and we were free to head home to Arkansas to our girls. We packed our bags, headed to the airport, and headed home with a bright outlook on the future we would have together as a family. I spent another week really recovering before I went back to work. I was feeling almost 100% at about 3-4 weeks, though still very careful about my activities. At about six weeks post surgery, I felt fine, and I was back to 100% activity level.

My husband and I began trying to conceive as soon as my recovery was complete. The first month went by and we had been unsuccessful. April came and went without a pregnancy. I began to read books on learning my body and the fertility signals it was giving me. I knew I had never had trouble getting pregnant before, but now everything was different. I was going to have to pay closer attention to my body and to what it was telling me if I was going to get pregnant after my tubal reversal. I began charting my BBT (basal body temperature) and recording on charts and graphs all of my other fertility signs. Then came May. On May 31, 2004, just three and a half months after my surgery, I received the best news any reversal patient could hope for. I got a positive pregnancy test! I called my local OBGYN to begin all the pregnancy tests he could possibly come up with. This was it! We were living our dream! I was pregnant with our child! The surgery had worked! We were so excited and anxious to meet this little one growing inside of me. I had an appointment two days later to begin my blood work so we could monitor the pregnancy.

Unfortunately, the news from the blood work was not good. The numbers were too low to indicate a normal pregnancy. The doctor wanted me to come back in three days to have more blood work done to see if the numbers would get better. We would have to wait and see if this would be a viable pregnancy. Three days later, I returned to the clinic to have more blood drawn. We found out the numbers were not rising, and this was not a viable pregnancy. Our world came crashing down around us. I miscarried on our one year wedding anniversary. We were crushed.

We were devastated at the loss of our first pregnancy, but encouraged that I was able to get pregnant so soon after my reversal. We began again to chart my fertility signs and trying to conceive right away. We couldn't believe it when we got another positive pregnancy test in August 2004. We were very excited about this pregnancy, yet cautious. We were still hurting from our loss. I couldn't imagine going through that again. I had my first blood work done on August 13, 2004. The report was good. The numbers from my blood work came back very solid. It looked like this pregnancy was going to make it. We were very happy, yet guarded. I continued my blood tests and the numbers continued to rise. We made our appointment for our first ultrasound August 23, 2004. That was one of the most difficult days to wait for. I wanted to know if this baby was going to make it. I wanted to know if we were going to be able to have this child we waited so long and worked so hard for. I had the weight of the world on my shoulders going into this ultrasound. When I saw that little pulsing heart on the monitor for the first time, I couldn't do anything but lay there and cry. There it was, our baby, our child.

My pregnancy was very uneventful with no problems to report whatsoever. On November 12, 2004, my husband adopted my two older daughters. On November 19, 2004, we discovered via ultrasound we were going to add yet another girl to our household! My husband was very overwhelmed, but you could already see this little girl wrapping her daddy around her tiny little finger.

Riley Alyse was born at 38 weeks gestation on April 5, 2005, at 1:10 p.m., after 7 hours of labor. She weighed 7lbs., 2oz., and was 20 ¾ inches long. She was perfectly beautiful and very healthy. To this day she is a perfect baby. We couldn't have asked for anything closer to an angel. We are planning on trying for a second reversal baby within the next couple of years.

Elaine's Journey
Chapter 11

What struck me about Elaine's story is the importance she placed on how precious the gift of life was. Elaine and her husband seem to have it all, by the standards of our society, but it wasn't enough. She longed for what is genuine. Her story is a perfect example of how material things are not the key to true happiness. Elaine was willing to give it all to have a child, even if it meant her sight. Here is Elaine's story.

When my first husband and I were still married, we decided to have the surgery to get my tubes tied. We had a boy and a girl together, and we wanted them to have the best of everything. Since we had our pair, we decided a tubal ligation would be best. We got a divorce soon after. I discovered that he had fathered two other children. I was devastated that his baby making days were not over, but mine were. I longed to have another child. At first, I thought it was just my hormones raging for another baby, but soon I was overwhelmed with thoughts and feelings for another. I met and eventually married my second husband, Victor. We lived a whirlwind life, going out, super terrific vacations, nice gifts, etc. But it wasn't enough. I still wanted another baby. Victor took good care of me and my two kids, and I knew he would make an excellent father. But he was scared to pursue that part of life. His childhood with his father was not the best. Eventually, my husband and I decided if it was meant to be, then it would happen.

I began researching tubal reversals on the internet. At first, I felt very overwhelmed with all the information from the internet about the reversal procedure. Then, I felt in control, and able to sort it all out and decide on a doctor. My husband was still scared, but we talked a lot about the procedure and possible positive outcome of the procedure. We researched together and spoke with Dr. Berger and his office, and we went over all the information. I am in the medical field, so I naturally asked a lot of questions. Then we realized insurance was not going to pay for it. So we had to figure out how we would come up with the money. We decided to use our yearly income tax refund that comes around Valentine's Day. I couldn't wait, so we took out a loan around Christmas time and had the tubal reversal late January 2003. I was scared how my family was going to react to my wanting to start over again with another baby. Everyone was for it, for the most part. I did have some people say I was crazy, but once I make up my mind, nothing can change it.

One of my biggest concerns before having the reversal, was my ability to be a good mom. My other two children were teenagers. Once I expressed my concerns to family and friends, they helped me to realize how wonderful my kids turned out. Once pregnant, because of my age, I would have to do things differently, for example, amniocentesis. This was difficult for me because I do not like needles.

Actually, I am terrified of them. But I knew I had to put my baby first and me last. I also had a medical condition called PTC (pseudo tumor cerebri) which is a benign condition that causes severe headaches and vision problems. Some of the doctors were afraid that the excess fluid from carrying a baby, and the hormones, would cause more problems along with the PTC. I could have lost my vision, and I would have to take meds during the pregnancy that could harm the baby. I suffered daily with this condition and was on different medications. Together with my OBGYN, family practice doctor, and my neurologist, I decided to take my chances and try to get pregnant. After I found out I was pregnant, the headache and vision problems stopped immediately.

Believe it or not, I knew I was pregnant the moment I conceived. Everything tasted different, and I felt like I was on cloud nine. I hadn't missed a period yet and had about two weeks before I could test to see if I was. I told everyone I was pregnant before the blood test even confirmed it. They all had about two weeks to absorb the news before the test confirmed it.

Everyone was amazed and overjoyed that the tubal reversal procedure worked. My husband and I were very happy and thankful. It was a great experience for us. My family was excited that we were going to have a baby. It had been a long time since the family had a baby around. My kids were especially happy. They kept up with the milestones of the pregnancy, often asking questions about how big the baby was, or how much it weighed.

Our due date was May 14, 2004. Baby Victor L., Jr. arrived on April 23, 2004, at 9:51 a.m., and weighed in at 7 lbs., 7.7 oz., lucky number 7-7-7. He was 20 inches long and in perfect health. He is our miracle baby, our angel, our true gift from God, and he is so loved. There are no words that can do justice to describe how I felt when my son was born. I was in awe of him, the way he looked, the way he smelled. I call him my precious angel, my love, because that's what he is. He was a gift sent to us, and we are truly blessed.

I can't begin to thank Dr. Berger and the staff enough for the miracle procedure that gave me my son. It has been a wonderful experience. The surgery was easy. I had it done on a Monday, recuperated on Tuesday, and took a tour of Graceland on Thursday on our way back to Texas. I would do it all again in a heartbeat.

Tori's Journey
Chapter 12

What I learned from Tori's story is to be persistent, it pays off. Although told a reversal was impossible and pressured to have in-vitro fertilization, Tori did not give up and did not take no for an answer. Because of that, she found Dr. Berger, and had a successful surgery that was said to be impossible. Here is Tori's story.

I got pregnant with twin boys when I was 23 years old. My first husband and I thought long and hard about getting my tubes tied after this. We came to an agreement that the twins were all the children he and I wanted together. We were happy with our decision, and my tubes were tied in October 1996. The surgeon that performed the tubal ligation put a ring on the right tube. The left tube ripped, so it was cut and burned.

The next year, my husband and I separated. The twins were now two years old. I began seeing the love of my life, my present husband John. He had no biological children of his own, and we wanted children together. He knew I had a tubal ligation, and it would be costly for us to have a baby. But he did not care. We told our primary doctor that we wanted to try to have a baby, but my tubes were tied.

I was sent to get a test to see if my tubes could be open before anything would be done. I was told they could not. We went to see an in-vitro specialist here in Michigan, but he seemed to be more about money for himself, than a baby for us. We were going to go ahead with it anyway. They told us they would call with a surgery date in a few days. John and I were so happy to finally get the ball rolling. Then they called. No appointment was set. Instead, they wanted us to send them the money. We were told it could actually take a few months to a year for a surgery date, and they would not be able to get a surgery date until the price was paid in full. Meanwhile, our estimated $10-$20,000 would be collecting interest in their bank, while we impatiently waited for a surgery date. A few months to a year was too long a wait for us. We decided we would not trust my body, or our baby with this doctor and his office.

Now mind you, all of this small stuff we were doing was taking time, lots of it. It seemed like forever between appointments, finding out tests results, and switching to different doctors. By now, I had done my pap tests, breast exams, blood work, and hysteropenogram.

I went back to my OBGYN. She sent us to another doctor about an hour from our home. We sat in her office about half and hour with no word, when finally a woman comes in and says, "The doctor wants you to stay and get a pap smear and breast exam done by her." Okay, they have the results from my doctor's office with the same tests I just had done a month ago. This new doctor, I had not even met yet, wants to do all her own testing. Apparently, she doesn't trust my doctor, the one who referred me to her. My insurance company pays for my regular appointments, but we have to pay out-of-pocket for anything we do in regards to trying to have a baby, since my tubal ligation was voluntary. We left her office.

Maybe a few months later, my mother-in-law calls us about a fertility specialist in North Carolina that my aunt heard about. My husband's aunt lives in North Carolina. His name, Dr. Gary Berger. I called his office and spoke with Rhonda. I asked her questions, she answered honestly. I told her the whole story from the beginning and all that we have done so far. A few days later, a video came in the mail explaining the surgery from the woman's perspective, as well as the man's. The video showed the surgery from beginning to end. I called and made an appointment. Within two weeks, we were on our way to Chapel Hill. Finally, something was happening, something that could actually help to make our baby. I was getting a tubal reversal!

We met with Dr. Berger for the first time in March 2000. Talk about an angel's face. He was so understanding and caring. He genuinely cared, about us, not the money he was making. He was able to reverse my right tube, however, the left tube was too short. Nevertheless, our dream became possible. After the surgery, I felt good. The surgery went just like the video said, no surprises. Dr.

Berger even removed scarring from my previous surgeries. I went home to Michigan the next day after my surgery.

A week after I returned home, Dr. Berger's office called to check on me. Life went on normally for me for about a year, wondering each month if this would be the month I would achieve a pregnancy. I did not become pregnant by this time, so I went to get checked. I found out that my cervix only had a small opening. I had surgery to laser it back open. They did another hysterpenogram, and my right tube was still open. We tried for another two years. It was now 2004. My OBGYN still only recommended in-vitro fertilization. Dr. Berger recommended getting my progesterone checked before spending the kind of money it took for in-vitro. My now ex-OBGYN would not do the testing. I felt as though he was making some kind of finders-fee to recommend in-vitro to his patients. I found another OGBYN that was recommended by my husband's cousin. I had finally found a great OBGYN, that is as caring as Dr. Berger. He checked my progesterone and it came out great. He decided to do a post-coital test next.

The same week I got the post-coital test done, I conceived. I found out I was pregnant on October 23, 2004, three days before I turned 32. My dream had come true. Of all the ways I considered telling my husband the great news, the only thing I could come up with was to go downstairs and hand him the test. For almost four years, I thought of funny, romantic, smart, and goofy ways to tell my husband we were going to have a baby, and what do I come up with, handing him the test. He had me take two more tests to be sure. It could not have turned out more perfect. We immediately got on the phone and called our family and friends. It was a great moment!

Our son is now 14 months old. He has two older brothers that love him and play with him. He has them to look up to. All my sons are my pride and joy. We are now trying to conceive again, and we are hoping for a girl. Of course, another boy would be great, too.

Within this whole period of time, four years, Dr. Berger and his staff were with me until I reached my pregnancy goal. There were phone calls between doctors in my own state, and phone calls to Dr. Berger instead of to those in my own state. If it weren't for Dr. Berger and his staff, I would still be trying to find a doctor that took the time to care. I may have even been going through in-vitro and other procedures and tests. Without Dr. Berger, we would not have our Ashton Hugh. I could never thank him enough for all he has done.

Never stay with a doctor you cannot trust, or do not feel comfortable with, and always have hope and faith. My husband and I drove to North Carolina from Michigan, paid for a hotel, had surgery out of state, and drove home in three days. We paid less money including our surgery, travel, and long distance calls to Dr. Berger than it would have cost us to have surgery in our own state. Best of all, it was less stressful with a doctor who is more qualified by doctors' standards, and over qualified by human standards.

Psalm 113:9

He settles the barren woman in her home as a happy mother of children. Praise the Lord!

Denise's Journey
Chapter 13

Denise heard of Dr. Berger through a neighbor she had befriended. I am amazed at how God puts others in our lives for reasons such as these. Had their paths not crossed, Denise may not have had a reversal and been blessed with two beautiful reversal babies.

My name is Denise Martell. I am a mother of five. Two of my children are tubal reversal babies. My reversal was done my Dr. Berger. When I was 23 years old, I had a tubal ligation after I had my third child. Two years later, I separated from my husband and divorced. I met a wonderful man who loved children, but did not have any of his own. After we were together a couple years, I called the doctor who did my tubal ligation to find out if my ligation could be reversed, but she did not do the reversal procedure. I called around and found a few doctors in the area that performed the reversal, but it would cost over $20,000. There was no way we could afford it, so we gave up on the idea.

About a year later, I made friends with the new neighbors. We got to talking about how we had both had our tubes tied, and how we both wished to have more children. I told her how we had called around to get a reversal, but we could never afford it. She told me she also looked into the procedure on the internet, and she came across a doctor in North Carolina named Dr. Gary Berger. She showed me the website. After reading everything, I showed it to my fiance. He was skeptical at first, so I sent them an e-mail and got a quick response. We took a few months to think about it and to make sure this is what we wanted to do. I had just turned 30, and my youngest child just turned eight at the time we decided to go ahead with the surgery. I got back in touch with Dr. Berger's office to find out what I needed to do, and if it was even possible for me to have a tubal reversal. I sent them the files they needed. After some slight confusion, we got everything straightened out and ready to go. I got the needed blood work completed, and I made an appointment to have a reversal.

My parents went with me because my soon-to-be husband could not get off work. We arrived at Dr. Berger's office on a Thursday morning. They were the friendliest people I think I have ever met. While waiting, we talked with the receptionists and looked at the photo albums of all the babies born after a reversal at Chapel Hill. I met with the nurses and had some tests done. Next, I got to speak with Dr. Berger. He was great!

I arrived the next morning for surgery. After making sure I was okay, I was sent to my hotel room where I slept the rest of the day. In the morning, Dr. Berger and a nurse came to my hotel room to see how things were going. I got the okay to go back home. I was told to take it easy for a few days, but didn't listen. I went shopping that day on the way back to Maine, and was coaching my daughter's softball team once home. I overdid it and was sore a lot longer than what I should have been.

On June 29th, I was married. Exactly nine months later on March 29, 2002, we had a beautiful baby boy. Thirteen months after that, on May 11, 2004, we had another boy. They would not be here if it weren't for the skill of Dr. Berger and his staff. I would recommend him to anyone who is thinking of having this done. My husband loves his stepchildren, but there is nothing like having a child call you daddy. We can't imagine what life would be like without these two little boys.

Hebrews 11:11,12

By faith Abraham, even though he was past age-and Sarah herself was barren-was enabled to become a father because he considered himself faithful who had made the promise. And so from this one man, and he as good as dead, came decendants as numerous as the stars in the sky and as countless as the sand on the seashore.

Melissa's Journey
Chapter 14

Melissa has what some of us online call post tubal syndrome. Some say there is no proof of this, but many women claim to have terrible side effects after tubal ligation. Many women seek a reversal to reverse the damage caused to their health by a tubal ligation. Being given one of God's little ones to care for is an added bonus. Here is Melissa's story.

I knew almost from the time I had my tubal ligation that it was a big mistake. I began having a lot of bleeding and severe pain, often twice a month. At the time of my ligation, I was still in a violent marriage which I felt made the decision to have a tubal ligation a necessity. Five years later, I ended that marriage and began to rebuild my life, and the lives of my two older children. Two years later, beating the odds, I remarried a wonderful man. My health had deteriorated drastically due to the pain and excessive bleeding. We talked with doctors locally and scheduled my surgery with my OBGYN, whom I'd known for many years. Now at this time, I knew of Dr. Berger, but was reluctant to travel that far to have surgery with a doctor I didn't know. After going into laparoscopy, my doctor determined the damage to my tubes to be too extensive to repair. We paid for a procedure that wasn't able to be performed. He suggested we try in-vitro fertilization to conceive, but we thought the success rate wasn't very good, and we weren't just trying to conceive, we were trying to put my body back together again.

After much thought, prayer, and financial juggling, we scheduled surgery with Dr. Berger. Everyone there was so kind; from Melanie who did a lot of the initial set up and paperwork, to Patti who followed up afterwards. Dr. Berger was confident that even with 2 cm of tube on one side, 6 cm on the other, and only one ovary as well, that we should be able to conceive. He was right! Just over a year later, while on a family camping trip, I was late. I took an HPT and it was positive. When we got home, further testing was done to ensure the pregnancy wasn't ectopic. Everything was fine. Other than some illness during pregnancy, which is normal for me, everything went well.

James Brannon Nunamaker was born at 6:00 p.m. on April 22, 2004. At 8lbs., 15oz., he was my biggest baby yet, but oh how welcome once he arrived. He is now his big brother and sister's joy and sorrow as he follows them everywhere and gets in their stuff. He is my husband's first biological child, so Daddy James has had to learn to put away his things as well. What changes such a little person brings? We couldn't imagine life without him. Now he just needs a little sister to go along with him.

Keri's Journey
Chapter 15

I imagine a lot of women, after being told a reversal is out of the question, would just give up and go on. Luckily, in Keri's case, she didn't take no for an answer and ended up with a beautiful blessing because of it. Here is Keri's story.

I have two sons from a previous marriage, Clint, 16, and Justin, 10. When their dad and I got divorced, I decided to have my tubes tied. I was done. Well, Mr. Wonderful entered my life in November, 2001. He had no children of his own. I figured he didn't want any either because he had none of his own from a previous 14 year relationship. I was wrong. He told me he did, but my tubes were tied. He told me from the get go that he knew they could be reversed somehow. But the first thing we did was have a sperm analysis completed to make sure everything was okay there.

We got married in June 2003. I set out to find a doctor soon after. I found one in my state, and set up an appointment with him. I had one visit with him and was very uncomfortable. He basically told me my chances on having a successful reversal were slim to none. The cost was very expensive, too. I came home and told my husband I was uncomfortable with the doctor and did not want to use him. My husband then went online and found

Dr. Berger. It sounded great, but I was hesitant because I don't like to fly. But after talking to Dr. Berger's staff, I knew Dr. Berger would be the best choice for us. We had the surgery in May 2004.

My menstrual cycle began again right after the surgery. We tried that first month for a pregnancy, but nothing. In July, our second month trying to conceive, something just felt different. I took an HPT, and surprisingly, it was positive. I could not believe it was positive so soon. I was so excited! I went to my husband's job site to tell him. He was thrilled, too!

So here starts the beginning of nine long months. We had an ultrasound at 16 weeks. We put up wagers on whether it was a boy or girl. My husband said boy, I said girl. My husband and two sons were there during the ultrasound to find out we were having a baby boy. The look on my husband's face, I will never forget. He was having a son. The boy's were very happy, too.

My due date was March 8, 2004. That day came and went. I was induced on the 15th of March. After a long day, my son arrived at 7:55 p.m. The actual labor was not long, about an hour. My husband was so incredible throughout the whole process. Then to see my little one. What can I say? I never pictured myself with a new little one, and here he was, so beautiful and tiny. We bonded right away. He is my Patrick Kevin. He is so loved and much wanted.

Patrick is now 5 ½ months old and is such a big boy. We have this overwhelming gift of life. I am so glad my husband is able to experience fatherhood with his own child. He is so good with my two older boys, so I knew he'd make a great dad. We are now working on reversal baby two.

We are forever grateful to Dr. Berger and his staff. I thank God for making all this happen. We are forever grateful for our "slice of heaven, Patrick Kevin."

Psalm 37:4

Delight yourself in the Lord and he will give you the desires of your heart.

Christy's Journey
Chapter 16

Christy is one of many examples of women getting pregnant with only one tube. There are many women out there who have done the same. Have hope, it does happen. Here is Christy's story.

Unlike most tubal reversal candidates, I have not been divorced, or been remarried to a man that doesn't have children of his own. I felt really alone when I first decided to have a reversal because I didn't know anyone else like me who was seeking this procedure. A lot of people judged me for having a tubal ligation in the first place. I felt in our current situation it was the right thing to do. We were struggling with our house payment. Knowing I would want more children, but not wanting to make things harder on my husband, I had a tubal ligation. That was in 1998. I had one son and one daughter. Everyone thought I should be happy with that. That decision turned out to be a huge mistake. I suffered a terrible case of the baby blues after my daughter was born due to my decision to get my tubes tied. It added strain to my marriage, too. I also began to have a lot of medical problems such as periods lasting about three weeks, and a week later, starting again with the same. I ended up in the hospital a few times with horrible cramps and severe bleeding. My doctor stated my ligation did not cause this, but after researching the internet, I found many women who experienced the same symptoms as I did after their tubal ligations.

In 2001, our financial status had changed. We decided to have a reversal. We still had to come up with the money and tell my family who thought I was crazy for wanting more kids when I already had a boy and girl. We borrowed money against my husband's Thrift Savings Plan, so that we would just be paying ourselves back. It was taken right out of his check, so we didn't even miss the money.

We made the trip to Chapel Hill from West Virginia. We met the staff the night before the surgery, and we met Dr. Berger, too. By other doctor's standards, I was too overweight to be considered for surgery, but not with Dr. Berger. I was so excited to have a doctor who didn't look at me for my weight, or request a picture of my body in a swimsuit as some do. Dr. Berger stated that the reversal would probably help with all the horrible symptoms I was having since the ligation. At least if the Lord didn't bless us with any more children, I would as least be well enough to take care of the children I now have. The surgery went well. I do not remember my tube lengths. I do know they weren't great, but good.

The following morning, one of the nurses came by to check on me. After leaving, my family and I took a mini vacation to Virginia Beach. We had a great time, and I did not have much pain. I just had to rest a little after long walks on the beach, but other than that, I recovered great.

We started trying to conceive right away in August. In December, after no pregnancy, I went to have an HSG done to see if the tubes remained open. I knew there was a possibility they could close because sometimes it just happens. Well, one tube was blocked. I was devastated. I went to a fertility specialist and found out I was not ovulating. I was prescribed Clomid, and I finally got pregnant with my reversal angel, Noah Robert, with only one tube. Noah was born January 28, 2003. He was such a miracle! We were so happy to have another little one in our lives.

After Noah's birth, I ended up gaining more weight. I decided to have gastric bypass surgery in April 2004. I lost over 100 lbs., and was soon pregnant with our second reversal baby. Little Isaiah was born on July 5, 2005. He is doing great and is now 8 weeks old. We are thinking about trying for a little girl, but will take a little boy, too, of course. We love our big family. I get tons of weird looks from people when they see how many kids we have, or the ones who ask when we are going to stop having children because they think we have enough. But to us, they are our little angels. God placed them in our lives for a reason as we see it. We just try to give them all the love they need, and we always get lots back.

I will always thank Dr. Berger for never judging me in the first place for getting my tubes tied, and for the mere fact that he did the surgery without any regards to my weight. Dr. Berger and his staff were very wonderful and supportive.

1 John 5:14,15

This is the confidence we have in approaching God: that if we ask anything according to his will, he hears us-whatever we ask-we know that we have what we asked of him.

Lori's Journey
Chapter 17

Faith, hope, and patience played a major factor in the lives of Lori and her husband. They were set on the promise that God would deliver His blessings, in His own timing, and if His will. Here is Lori's story.

Dr. Berger performed my tubal reversal for me in May 2001. My husband and I sought the reversal after the death of our four year old daughter, Katie, in February 2001, from a very sudden Group A Strep infection. We had a tubal ligation after her birth because she was intended to be an only child. Within weeks of this, we knew we had to place the decision of future children back into the hands of God.

My husband is turning 44, and I just turned 41 this past January. We knew that if we were meant to have another child, it would be totally up to the Lord, without any fertility treatments to help us along. I got pregnant in July 2001, but miscarried in October, at approximately ten weeks into the pregnancy. I knew that this miscarriage came with a message. Everything within me and my husband was functioning fine, and a child, if one was to come, would come in God's timing, not ours. Our job was to be patient and wait on His timing. The past four years since our reversal have not been in vain. We have healed so much from the loss of our Katie. I believe that was all a part of God's timing, which is perfect for us in so many ways now.

As of this writing, I am currently 32 weeks pregnant due with our son in 6-8 weeks. I wanted to share our wonderful news, and to thank Dr. Berger for the part he and his staff at Chapel Hill played in helping to lead us to this blessing. I know that the birth of this precious child will always give me the opportunity to give credit to the skills of Dr. Berger and to waiting on the Lord. We feel that when we began searching the internet and asking questions of my OBGYN about getting a tubal reversal, there were definite signs from God that we were to seek the help of Dr. Berger instead of any other doctor. I truly know that the Lord has been guiding us since Katie's death. I knew I could trust him to guide the surgery, in addition. Getting pregnant in 2001 was proof that the surgery was a success, and a wonderful job had been done. Time was the only ingredient needed, although it was the hardest to tolerate. I thank Dr. Berger for choosing this ministry to all those families that seek God's most precious gifts.

Bella's Journey
Chapter 18

I really appreciate the honesty and sincerity of Bella's story. She's had some good times and some bad times, and maybe even made some unwise choices, but in her faith, she made it through and trusted God to provide his blessings. After one tube to work with, three years of trying to conceive, and time against her, God saw her through. I hope her story will convince you that nothing is impossible with God. Here is Bella's story.

My story is one I would love for someone to read who is considering having a tubal ligation, to possibly change their mind. To begin, I was happily married. We had a boy in 1984 and a girl in 1986, which we thought was a wonderful family, having one of each. Times were rough financially, and we were living with my parents at the time. My first husband couldn't seem to keep a job, only seasonal work, or he was getting hurt at work. I did not want to burden my parents. I thought having a tubal ligation would be a good idea, so I had it done. Then came the bad news. Women started calling for child support. There were many of them. He walked out on us for a while. It took some time, but he did come back. I had two little ones and wanted them to have both their mom and dad together to raise them. So we tried to make things work, but he was continuously unfaithful.

Things later began to turn around in my life. I met someone wonderful, someone who treated me like a woman and who only wanted to be with me. He was nine years younger than I. I was 29 when we met, and he was just turning 21. John and I got an apartment, and after five years together, we took off and got married. We drove to Niagra Falls, NY, and were married in a wedding gown and tuxedo along the Bridal Veil Falls on September 9, 1999. John knew I could never have children and married me anyway.

The time came when we started wanting children together. I asked my former sister-in-law to think about becoming a surrogate mother, and carry our child for us. She had already given two previous children up for adoption. I asked my OBGYN if my tubes could be fixed and opened, and his answer was no, it was a permanent procedure. I went for a second opinion. I was told it would cost at the minimum $10,000. That was just for the doctor's bill. This did not include hospitalization and medications, and all with no guarantee the reversal would even work. I was actually told there was a 90% chance that the procedure wouldn't work.

From there, I decided to look on the internet for whatever information I could dig up. I found several doctors and support groups by typing tubal reversal in my search engine. Dr. Berger caught my attention. I called the office and later sent him all the paperwork pertaining to my tubal ligation. I had also spoken with two other doctors, but easily decided on Dr. Berger. I knew in my heart of hearts, he would be the best choice for me. His success rate was extraordinary, he was close to home, and the cost of the surgery was very reasonable. He offered a discount to support group ladies if some of us scheduled together on the same day. I turned in my retirement plan to pay for the surgery and scheduled it for August 15, 2000.

On our way to Chapel Hill, we stopped in Virginia Beach to meet two of the ladies from one of my reversal support groups. They shared their reversal stories and some great advice. When we arrived in Chapel Hill, we had our consultation with Dr. Berger, and we got to meet the staff. We looked through album after album of babies who were born to women who had their reversals with Dr. Berger. There were many! I could tell I was in the hands of a very experienced doctor. Surgery would be the next morning. As we waited in the waiting area, we talked with other men and women there, most with stories just like mine. The stories were similar-women who regretted having a tubal ligation, women who had a ligation for others, those who had a ligation because they were in a bad relationship, and those who married a man who had no children of their own.

We showed up for surgery the next morning. About all I remember is talking to a nurse, seeing a needle, and I was out. It took me a long time to come out of it, longer than most. My husband John was beginning to worry. He was already more worried about surgery than I had been. But it all turned out fine. There hadn't been anything wrong but a bad case of nausea, wanting to vomit and feeling very weak. I had some sort of electronic device with a control that would turn the vibration up or down. It was used to stimulate the incision and help it heal faster. I was informed that the surgery went great, but I had only one reversible tube. The doctor who performed my tubal ligation cut out the fimbria end of the right tube. Now I know why the doctor who performed the tubal ligation said "uh-oh." He had accidentally cut where he shouldn't have. He had not told me this, or added it into the operative report. I guess he figured I wouldn't want more children anyway, so why worry about it. I felt my chances to conceive another child were cut in half now. I was already 37 when I had the reversal and felt time was against me, too.

We tried and tried for one year with no medications, or any form of testing. I had medical insurance that would pay for one year of infertility treatments, but I had a long fight and appeals because they wanted to disqualify me due to the fact that I had a tubal ligation to begin with. Even though they did not pay for the reversal, they would not help me with infertility issues.

We went on with some testing anyway. I have had many tests. I have had a test which measures the thickness of the uterus to see if an egg could implant, a dye test (HSG) twice to see if my tube was open or blocked because of scar tissue, and many others. A lot of the tests hurt, but I think we withstand a lot to have the gift of a beautiful child. My husband had a sperm analysis done twice. The test showed plenty of sperm, but slow motility rates.

I tried Clomid next, but that didn't work. My husband took about everything on the web that suggested it would improve the motility rate and quality of sperm. I had taken folic acid, baby aspirin, prenatal vitamins, Clomid, progesterone, etc. I even purchased a fertility monitor which is used to help forecast your most fertile days. Trying to conceive became a chore. We used every suggestion possible, and I had several tests which showed no reason why I couldn't conceive, but it just wasn't happening. This went on for a long stressful three years.

In March 2003, we both tried Fertility Blend for men and for women, which contain supplements that optimized female fertility and reproductive health. For men, it optimized sperm quality and fertility health. It recommend giving it three months to work it's way through the system. We couldn't take anymore. We gave up and just quit trying. We even considered foster care at one point just so we could have kids around.

The weekend of July 4, 2003, we went away for a four hour ride to my sister's house in Maryland. That night after the fireworks, we had finally conceived, although we didn't know it at the time. I think getting away together and not stressing over trying to conceive may have been the key. I suggest to others struggling with trying to conceive to just take a break, give up for a while, relax, and enjoy each other.

I am so blessed and so thankful to God! I prayed and prayed for my baby boy, and my prayers were answered! Maybe we were being tested, to see how much we would go through, whether we were worthy of the gift of a child. I don't know. But, good things come to those who wait. Read and write down John 14:14. Believe! He wants you to have that child! Believe it will happen, and ask Him in His name for that baby. I am sitting here with tears running down my face because I know I am so blessed. My little guy is so beautiful. He is now 18 months old. His older brother is 21, and his older sister is 19. He also has a foster brother who just turned eight. I am proof that God blesses you, he really does. I have been through so much good, yet so much bad, too. It's more than I can write about, but regardless, God blessed me on February 26, 2004 with a 5 lb. preemie, the day before I turned the big 4-0!

I thank Dr. Berger everyday. God used him to make our dreams come true. My husband can now experience the gift of having a child and someone to pass on his name. Our son's name is Andrew John William Myers, but we call him A.J. We honored a lot of relatives with his birth name.

My advice to all is to just relax, if it is God's will, it will happen. If you are reading this and are considering a tubal ligation, don't do it! Life changes! Leave children up to God! We are truly blessed by the almighty one!

Dolores' Journey
Chapter 19

I think you will appreciate Delores' story. Although she had so much going against her throughout this whole process, she has kept a positive outlook and has not given up, knowing that the Lord had a plan for her and her husband. She also gives hope for those trying to conceive out there who are "one-tubers", like herself, and is a perfect example of how God can work changes in our husbands when it comes to His blessings. Here is the journey of Delores.

My husband Eric and I were married in 1988. He was 17, and I had just turned 18. During the first five years of our marriage, we had 3 children. The year was 1993 when our decision was made to have a tubal ligation after the birth of our third son. Several weeks passed before I realized I had made a mistake. I was putting away the maternity clothes, blaming my new feelings on hormones, baby blues, whatever, I regretted the decision. I was only 23 years old and never going to be able to have babies again. I wanted a large family, but my husband Eric felt that three sons were more than we could handle at the time. I stuffed my misery away, promising Eric that three would be enough.

Over time, I began to distance myself from my husband, finally asking for a divorce in 1997. The decision to have the tubal ligation wasn't the only problem in our marriage, but I grew to resent him for it, even though I agreed to it. Fortunately, God had other plans for us. Shortly after I requested a divorce, Eric and I attended a Family Life Weekend to Remember Marriage Conference, where we were given the tools to help make our marriage work. During one of the exercises, I told Eric of the resentment I had towards him because of the tubal ligation. He was firm in his stance that three children were enough. I realized that God would have to change his heart, because I could not.

It was about then that I began looking into tubal reversal surgery, hoping to arm myself with information to present to Eric. Over the next six years, I sent operative reports to various doctors, all with discouraging results. I also received a lot of misguidance. One day, I found Dr. Berger in Chapel Hill, North Carolina. I sent in my operative reports, and was pleased to get a call the next day stating to me that I would be an excellent candidate for a tubal reversal. Now, I just had to get my husband on board. I had done a lot of praying and a lot of crying. I remember telling God I just wanted to be pregnant, to feel life within me one more time. I asked God to please help me once again talk to Eric.

In July 2003, I approached him about the surgery. He said to look into it, talk to Dr. Berger's office some more, and we'd talk about it later. Later turned into Eric needing more time to think about it. In February 2004, Eric spoke the words that were music to my ears. He said, "I think that if you are willing to go through the surgery, I would be honored to have another child with you." Crying, I hugged him, and told him how much I loved him.

In April 2004, I had the surgery with Dr. Berger. We traveled to Chapel Hill with great joy and hope in our hearts. The closer to the facility we got, the more nervous I got. Yet, the sheer excitement of finally being so close overcame the nervousness. We got to the surgical center and were greeted so warmly. We sat in the waiting room flipping through photo albums of babies that wouldn't have been alive if their mommies hadn't sat in the same room we were currently sitting in. Cathy came out to meet us, and she took us back for the usual pre-exam formalities and our ultrasound. Eric was in awe at the ultrasound, having never been with me when I had them done with the three boys. He was impressed with the professionalism and courtesy with which we were given. We met with Dr. Berger, and of course, we had our photo taken with him. Prior to leaving Pennsylvania, which is where we live, I had already started a scrapbook for our future child.

On April 6, 2004, Eric kissed me as I walked into the surgical suite. Waking up in recovery, the first thought on my mind was that I was fertile again. I looked at Eric standing over me, and cried, my heart bursting with joy at this man I almost lost. How amazing he was through it all! Dr. Berger came to talk to us, letting us know how the surgery went. There was nothing on the left side, as we had already known, due to the tumor I had removed 12 years prior, but the right side was 5.5 cm. Some very amazing news!

We waited out the new cycle and began trying to conceive in May 2004. Nothing happened that first cycle. On the second cycle, we watched for ovulation to approach and for my temperature to rise and stay there. I was amazed when my temperature continued to climb. I took an HPT and it was positive! I thought, oh my goodness, we are going to have a baby in March, just in time for my birthday. Our joy was short lived though. Three days later, I miscarried. My heart broke. We named our baby Isabella Grace.

We continued on for the next several months, hoping for a new pregnancy. I prayed as Hannah did in 1 Samuel for a child to dedicate and give back to the Lord. In November, my luteal phase was so short, only eight days. I called my OBGYN, and requested a progesterone level check. Sure enough, it was low. I then started Clomid, 50mg. It was successful in raising my progesterone level. Sadly, no pregnancy that month. On February 7, 2005, I started with my second cycle of Clomid. Isabella's due date was here on March 4, 2005. Eric stayed home with me to comfort me in my grief. He realized it was time for me to test, but I refused. Over the weekend, he asked me if I had tested with an HPT. On Sunday morning, March 6th, I tested. I could not believe my eyes. It was positive. I crawled back into bed and kept my secret until we were in church later that day. I opened my Bible to 1 Samuel 1:27 where

Hannah had thanked God for her son. "For this child I prayed and the Lord has granted me my petition which I asked of Him." I handed my Bible to Eric. After a few moments, he realized what I was trying to tell him.

On March 14, 2005, I awoke from a dream where a little boy, who looked like my youngest son, came to me and said, "I have to go now mommy. I love you." I went to the bathroom and discovered I was bleeding. Cavan Charles went to heaven on the wings of an angel that morning.

We later found out I have a problem with blood clots because my body isn't able to absorb folic acid properly. Currently, I take high doses of folic acid daily, in addition to B6 and B12. Clomid is still part of my monthly regime, at least until October. We added Estradiol, too.

Do I now regret having a tubal reversal, absolutely not! I would do it again in a heartbeat. To me, that surgery was a great success. I know my one tube is open, and that we time everything correctly. In this process, I have learned that God does keep his promises, but on his timetable, not mine. I can't thank Dr. Berger enough for making it possible for me to have this chance.

There are no words to express how much I owe Eric for being a strong pillar for me during this rollercoaster ride. He has held me, loved me, dried my tears, shared my joy and hopes, and he loved me through it all.

Isaiah 30:18

Yet the Lord longs to be gracious to you; he rises to show you compassion. For the Lord is a God of justice. Blessed are all who wait for him!

Kelli's Journey
Chapter 20

When I read Kelli's story, my mouth literally dropped. Kelli's story is unlike any I have heard in the past four years of my reversal research. Most of us had our tubal ligation after deciding we didn't want any more children, but Kelli, never had any to begin with. She had a tubal ligation as a means to prevent any pregnancies, ever. Here is her story.

Our tubal reversal journey is somewhat unique. My husband, Michael, and I had been married almost seven years, when after much thought and discussion, we made the decision not to have any children. It wasn't a decision that was made hastily. We spent many hours discussing what it would mean to have or not to have children in our lives. After the decision was made, we decided the best option for us would be for me to have a tubal ligation.

In June 1996, we discussed this option with the OBGYN I had at the time, and she was wiling to perform the surgery. Her biggest concern was to make sure we never wanted to be pregnant under any circumstances, and that we understood the procedure was "not reversible." So at the age of 26, having no children, and having never been pregnant, I had a tubal ligation. My laparoscopic surgery was routine with the exception that my left fallopian tube was banded (ring), and my right was Hulka clipped.

Apparently, the banding mechanism quit functioning in the middle of the surgery. After the surgery, life for us as a couple went on, still believing for several years to come, that being "childless by choice" was right for us.

It was just within the last several years that the decision we made began to really weigh upon my heart. After spending hours with the young children of close friends, I became convinced that we had made the wrong decision to have the tubal ligation. My husband, however, was not so sure. He loved spending time with our friends' children and our nephew, but he wasn't convinced that we needed our own.

I began searching the internet in 2002 for adoption agencies. Since we had the tubal ligation, I was certain adoption was our only choice and only chance at possibly having a child of our own. I spent countless hours researching international adoption and the agencies that specialized in this type of adoption. I read, and re-read the stories of adoptive parents and their journeys. With each passing day, I became more and more aware that I indeed wanted a child of my own.

Out of curiosity, while researching on the internet, I went to a search engine and typed in tubal reversal. One of the sites it brought my attention to was the Chapel Hill Tubal Reversal Center and Dr. Berger. I immediately went to and read the entire site. I was very interested and requested one of the free videotapes of Dr. Berger performing the tubal reversal surgery. I continued to do research on tubal reversals, as well as the international adoption. I even contacted my new OBGYN and inquired about having one of their doctors perform the surgery. I was told that the surgery was difficult, expensive ($20,000), and would not necessarily be a success. I was devastated. I was sure that if I was going to have the surgery, it should be my own doctor performing it instead of a doctor I found on the internet. The cost was also prohibitive. It was almost as much as an international adoption, and there was no guarantee it would work.

I finally made a decision and submitted my tubal ligation operative report to Chapel Hill. Dr. Berger's staff called and told me I would be a good candidate for a reversal surgery. I was elated! However, I still had to convince my husband. I talked to him off and on about the options available to us. He would listen, ask questions, and promise to think about it. The convincing would take much prayer and several years. One day, while at church, I told him I know that we are meant to have at least one child, and that I wanted to pursue the international adoption. He replied that he knew I would want to have more than one, so why didn't we just have the tubal reversal surgery, so that if successful, we could have more than one child. I was thrilled!

I called Chapel Hill immediately and set up our appointment for surgery in January 2004. Once the appointment was set and everything was set into motion, my husband became very excited and involved. I continued to do research. However, now my focus was on trying to conceive. I read every book and magazine I could get my hands on. I also spent countless hours reading discussion boards on the internet. We began monitoring my cycles even before my surgery. I purchased computer software to record my temperatures and develop a sense of what my cycles were like and what my body was telling me when I was ovulating, hoping to make getting pregnant easier.

We arrived in Chapel Hill for surgery in January 2004. The staff of Chapel Hill Tubal Reversal Center were absolutely wonderful. The office staff, nurses, surgical staff, and especially Dr. Berger, treated us with so much care and compassion. Many of the nurses were shocked to find out that my husband and I had been married to each other for 14 years at the time, had never been pregnant, and that neither of us had children, and had a tubal ligation. Apparently, we were the first statistic like that they had heard of. Our surgery went without any complications and was deemed very successful. My right fallopian tube measured 8 cm and the left measured 5 cm after surgery. I am a firm believer to this day that God had it planned for the banding instrument to quit during my tubal ligation, because the longer of the two tubes was the side that was Hulka clipped.

We wanted to conceive as soon as possible after surgery. We were anxious to see if the surgery had indeed been a success, and with each passing day we were more ready to become parents. I would venture to say that I became obsessed. As any woman who has ever tried to conceive over several months, or who has ever had to deal with infertility will tell you, it can take over your life, all aspects of it, the temperature taking, the charting, the two week wait, and the disappointment when your menstrual period shows up because you are just sure "this was the month." All of these things can make what should be an exciting and fun time, frustrating and difficult. I would watch numerous shows on pregnancy and birth on the Discovery Health Channel, I spent hours in discussion rooms with other women trying to conceive. I would cry and pray, hoping that it would soon be us that got to tell everyone we finally got our "big fat positive." But the time it took, and the disappointment each month, began to take its toll on us.

After waiting 5 months, we decided mostly for my sanity, it was time to have the HSG done to determine if my tubes were indeed open. It did not make sense to continue on like we had if my tubes were not open. We scheduled this for June 2004. The procedure was very uncomfortable, but over with quickly. I was told by the radiologist to go home and keep trying, as he had seen a great percentage of women get pregnant after having this procedure done.

On July 18, 2004, we finally got our positive pregnancy test. I had actually taken 3 or 4 tests in the days before that, getting the faint positive each time. We were stunned and thrilled! Our test was confirmed by my primary care physician the next day. Due to being a tubal reversal patient, I chose to have my obstetric care followed by my OBGYN. Because of the increased risk of ectopic pregnancy after tubal reversal surgery, I was quickly given an appointment for blood work and an early (5 week) ultrasound. This began what was to be several stressful days for us. My blood work showed that we were indeed pregnant, but the ultrasound was inconclusive as to whether or not there was a gestational sac in the uterus. Surprisingly, although stressed, I remained very confident that the pregnancy was not ectopic. This was confirmed a week later during another ultrasound. At 6 weeks, we saw the gestational sac exactly where it should be, and we saw the most beautiful sight, that of our baby's heartbeat. From that day forward, our pregnancy progressed normally. I did experience gestational hypertension and had to be put on bedrest for the last four weeks of the pregnancy, but otherwise it was a happy, healthy pregnancy.

On March 28, 2005, being two days overdue, we had our labor induced. After 20 plus hours of labor, our beautiful baby girl was born assisted by vacuum extraction, weighing a healthy 8lbs., 5 oz., and measuring 20 inches long. We were ecstatic to finally meet her and see her beautiful face. To this day, as we look at her and watch her grow, it is hard to believe she is actually ours. She is the absolute joy of our lives. We know she is a miracle baby God has given to us, and in keeping with such, we dedicated her back to Him shortly after she was born. If it's God's will, we hope to start trying to conceive tubal reversal baby number two after Thanksgiving this year.

Our reversal journey has indeed been a life changing experience with the arrival of our precious daughter. I believe all things happen for a reason, and God has had His hand on our lives this entire time. I know He lead us to Chapel Hill and Dr. Berger. Why we went the route we did having the tubal ligation in the first place, one may never know. Maybe it is for someone else to hear our story and to know they are not alone, and that there are tubal reversal success stories.

My advice to those seeking a possible tubal reversal, or those who have had tubal reversal surgery and are trying to get pregnant, is to first handle everything with prayer, have patience, do your research, and seek other tubal reversal sisters with a positive outlook to talk to. Our tubal reversal sisters can offer a wealth of support. This is an awesome journey. It can and will have its ups and downs, but if God chooses to bless you with a tubal reversal baby, it is so worth everything we must go through.

Psalm 127:3-5

Sons are a heritage from the Lord, children a reward from Him. Like arrows in the hands of a warrior are sons born in one's youth. Blessed is the man whose quiver is full of them. They will not be put to shame when they contend with her enemies in the gate.

Laurie's Journey
Chapter 21

Laurie's story is unusual in that right before her second marriage, she had her tubes tied, instead of the opposite, as so many seek. But as fate would have it, God worked on their hearts, and they sought a reversal.

My husband and I were married in 1995. I had two daughters from a previous marriage, ages 8 and 6, but he did not have any children of his own at the time. He was certain that he did not want any more children than the two I had, so we decided that I would have my tubes tied shortly before we were married. The doctor did a ligation with O rings.

In the fall of 2000, my husband suddenly decided he wanted to have a child of his own. This decision brought turmoil into our marriage because he thought that since my tubes were tied, there was no hope for him to have a child of his own. When he finally brought the problem to me, I spent a lot of time researching our options on the internet, and found that many women have had tubal reversal surgery with great success. I also wanted another child, so this was an easy decision for me.

We were both elated to find that there may be a solution to our situation, and began the process of finding a doctor. We initially chose a doctor about an hour and a half away from us. This doctor ordered numerous tests, none of which turned out to be necessary for the procedure. This became extremely expensive and time consuming, so I returned to Dr. Berger's website for further information regarding his procedures.

I became convinced that Dr. Berger was the answer to our prayers. I immediately called Dr. Berger's office and was given an appointment that was only two weeks away. We made the trip to Chapel Hill in the early part of April 2001. When we arrived at Dr. Berger's office, we were both very excited, but also apprehensive about the procedure. I was 35 years old at the time, but in good health. Dr. Berger and his staff were wonderful throughout the entire procedure. The surgery took place as scheduled, early in the morning, and we were back to our hotel room by noon.

I spent the rest of the day resting as ordered. Pain was no issue, as the pain unit Dr. Berger gave me was doing a wonderful job managing my pain. In fact, I did not feel much pain at all throughout my recovery. The next morning, Dr. Berger and his nurse came to our hotel room to check on me. After this short visit, we were given permission to make the eight hour trip home. Recovery from surgery was very easy. I was back to work that Monday with no discomfort whatsoever. We were hoping and praying each day that the procedure would work, and we would have a baby very soon.

By the beginning of June 2001, about 2 months

later, I was feeling a few pregnancy symptoms. I decided to take an HPT on Father's Day. My husband received the best Father's Day present ever that day. He was definitely going to be a new dad in February 2002. The look on his face when I told him the news was priceless. He couldn't wait to break the news to everyone we knew. He went to every doctor appointment with me, and was eagerly awaiting to learn the sex of our child through the amniocentesis my doctor had ordered. In September 2001, we learned that we were going to be blessed with a daughter.

Even though it had been 14 years since my last pregnancy and delivery, this pregnancy was the easiest and most enjoyable. On February 11, 2002, my water broke at 5:00 a.m. We arrived at the hospital before 6:00 a.m., and was induced at 8:00 a.m. since the contractions would not begin on their own. This did not alarm me as my second pregnancy delivered the same way. I was in labor all day with my husband close by. The best moment of all came at 8:37 p.m., when our daughter, Kelsey Marie, was born. Immediately after she was born, her proud father snatched her up in his arms. I will never forget the sight of him holding our daughter for the first time. This moment will forever be in my heart.

Kelsey will be 4 years old soon. She has been the light of our lives since the day she was conceived. She is a beautiful girl with blonde hair and bright blue eyes. She loves to read books, play with her Barbie dolls, and sing and dance to every song she hears. We thank God every day for sending us Dr. Berger. Without his help, we would not have been blessed with Kelsey. Dr. Berger is truly and angel who helps deliver miracles.

Having a tubal reversal was the best thing I have ever done in my life. My only regret is that I did not call Dr. Berger sooner. I tried a fertility doctor close to home and was disappointed with the results. The only thing that doctor had accomplished in four months was to order every expensive test available. My insurance would not cover these tests, and we ended up spending a great deal of money just to receive nothing in return. The day I found Dr. Berger's website was the day I knew in my heart that he was the answer to our prayers. He requested only a couple of blood tests and a copy of the tubal ligation post operative report. Surgery was scheduled quickly, and was completed as scheduled. He was very open and honest about the procedure, every step of the way, and we left there feeling confident that we would soon be pregnant. In fact, we were pregnant within two months of the surgery. If you are considering tubal reversal, you should make the trip to see Dr. Berger. I would refer anyone to him. Again, he is truly an angel who helps deliver miracles.

JoAnn's Journey
Chapter 22

After several long months of trying to conceive, JoAnn decided to take a break from trying. She became pregnant the month she did. Some say stress can play a factor in our ability to conceive. Another reason to let go, and let God work in our lives, under his timetable. Here is JoAnn's story.

My tubal reversal journey has taught me to never say never. We thought after having my tubes tied, we could never have another child. My husband and I had our first two children two years and three months apart. We knew that was all our lives could handle at that point in time, and a tubal ligation seemed to be a very sound decision.

But time changes everything. We reached a point in our lives when we knew we wanted another child. We were older and more mature, and hoped that we could slow down and enjoy a third pregnancy and child, more than we had allowed ourselves, or been capable of the first two times around. After twelve and a half years of marriage, and having children ages seven and five, we took the plunge and decided we could do diapers all over again.

My husband researched tubal reversal on the internet, and the information we found pointed us to

Dr. Berger in Chapel Hill, North Carolina. We live in Rome, Georgia, about an hour northwest of Atlanta.

Now, we did not have $6,000 just lying around, so we tried to creatively brainstorm about where this money was going to come from. We chose to cash out part of my 401K, as this was certainly as worthy an investment. We scheduled surgery for Thursday, May 30, 2002.

From the very first contact we had with Chapel Hill Tubal Reversal Center on the phone, asking questions and scheduling my surgery, I was quickly finding that this was the most courteous and professional medical office I had ever (and probably will ever) come in contact with. This proved to be true in my care before, during, and after my surgery. They continued to follow up on me even after I was home. They called six months after my surgery to see if I was pregnant yet and to see if I had any questions.

My surgery report from my tubal ligation revealed that my doctor had used the Pomeroy technique, and that he had found a hematoma on my right side when he was performing the tubal ligation. He cauterized this during the procedure. Dr. Berger was able to successfully repair both of my fallopian tubes. I had new tube lengths of 4 cm on the right and 4.5 on the left. I was disappointed that my tubes were not longer, but at least I had a chance to conceive.

When I returned home and began trying to conceive, I assumed it would happen quickly for me.

When I began my second cycle post reversal, I started temping and charting daily. I also added ovulation predictor kits to help with my efforts. As the 12th cycle post reversal loomed with still no pregnancy, I scheduled an HSG to see if my tubes were both still open. I must add that I truly believed that God would bless us with another child. I had hope and faith that he would make it happen. My HSG revealed that the right tube appeared to be at least partially blocked. But, the left side was wide open. We sent the films to Dr. Berger for review, and he agreed that it was not likely that I would be able to conceive from the right side. We also had a sperm analysis run on a sample from my husband to make sure that his part of the equation was okay. His test revealed that his levels were completely normal.

At that point, I asked my doctor for a prescription of Clomid. So many other women were trying it. I had learned a lot about it and other common fertility tricks being used. I was already ovulating every month and having normal cycles. But with only one tube, I figured why not? My doctor gave me a prescription for four months worth. My insurance would not cover this either, but it was only about twenty dollars a month. The only side effect that I experienced from the Clomid was severely decreased amounts of cervical mucus, including none of the egg-white cervical mucus so important during ovulation. Again, I emailed one of Dr. Berger's nurses, and in less than an hour, she replied with the name of an estrogen supplement drug to ask my doctor for. I took it the next month and sure enough, my cervical mucus returned. After three cycles of Clomid and still no pregnancy, I decided I needed a break from all trying to conceive efforts. I would just try not to think about it for a few months, and then dive in again, hopefully with renewed energy.

That first month on break, my 15th cycle, and fourteen months since my surgery, I was rewarded with my first positive pregnancy test. I had wasted so much money on pregnancy tests in those fourteen months that I had finally promised myself that I would not test until I was at least one day late for my period. A few days before my period was due, I noticed that I was extra tired and my breasts were very sore. I was having very mild off and on cramping and figured "Aunt Flo" must not be far away. The day my period was due, I felt mildly nauseous that entire day. I figured it was nerves due to getting my hopes up once again. But, just in case, I had a pregnancy test ready for in the morning. I caught my first morning urine with a cup, so that I would not waste a test. I opened the test kit and used the dropper to retrieve just the right number of drops to use on the test. I filled the test kit and left the bathroom to try and wait the full two minutes. I couldn't and went back to check. There was my double blue line on the pregnancy test! I told my husband and he did not believe me. I brought the test and showed it to him. He was in shock as much as I was.

I called my doctor's office as soon as they opened. I told them I had orders to have HCG levels drawn every 48 hours until I reached 1500, per Dr. Berger's protocol. They wrote the order accordingly. By lunchtime, I knew that my first level, at approximately 15 days past ovulation, was 125. I went exactly every 48 hours for my next draw, each time praying that my level would double properly. My second draw was 328. My third was 583. That was not a double. Did that mean something was wrong? Was I going to miscarry? It was a long 48 hours before my fourth and final draw was done and came back. But my fourth level more than tripled and came in at 2111. I scheduled my ultrasound for the next morning. My ultrasound revealed two sacs in the uterus. The positioning of one was high in the uterus exactly where it should be. The second sac had an odd shape to it and it's viability was questionable. We repeated the ultrasound seven days later. The first sac had grown and had a tiny heartbeat in it. The second sac had not grown and looked cloudy. The technician said, based on the heartbeat being 109, it had probably just started beating within the last 24 hours. Amazing!

I had a healthy pregnancy filled with lots of morning sickness and vomiting for the first seventeen weeks. Heartburn, indigestion, nasal stuffiness, and backaches were a few symptoms I had.

I thought I might be having a girl. The name we picked out was Grace Elizabeth. Grace has special significance for me, as this baby was a gift from God. It was through His amazing grace that I was pregnant. The ultrasound technician informed us, however, that we were expecting a baby boy. I turned to my husband and said, "Now we don't get to use Grace Elizabeth!" Then off the top of his head he replied, "What about Grayson?" We added Matthew as his middle name since it means "gift from God."

After two previous deliveries, I knew what to expect. I knew that due to the rod in my back from a previous surgery for scoliosis, my epidurals did not take properly. I researched alternatives to epidurals, such as spinal block. I talked to doctors and anesthesiologists about my options. I had been through labor and delivery with my sister who had an epidural that worked properly, and she was smiling and laughing and totally pain free throughout her whole delivery. It was amazing to me. I dreamed of being able to have the same.

Five days before my due date, my water broke on one of those many trips to the bathroom in the middle of the night. I arrived at the hospital dilated to a four, and with contractions 5 minutes apart. Since this was my third child, the newest nurse on the staff was assigned to me. I brought the x-rays of my spine with me and expressed my desire to have an epidural. Since it was the middle of the night, she didn't want to wake either the OBGYN, or the anesthesiologist. She waited too long. Less than three hours later, I was ready to push. I gave birth, completely natural, to my beautiful baby boy. Grayson Matthew weighed 7lbs., 14 oz. and was 19 inches long.

The joy he has brought to our lives is indescribable. His older brother and sister simply adore him as well. They are not jealous at all, and know that he was meant to be a part of our family. Grayson has been such a blessing that we are now considering a fourth addition to the family. Once he reaches his second birthday we might give it a try. Our tubal reversal journey has enriched our lives in so many ways. Where we chose to have the surgery has greatly influenced the entire experience. I thank God for my amazing gift and for sending me to Chapel Hill and Dr. Berger's office.

1 Samuel 1:27

I prayed for this child, and the Lord has granted me what I asked of Him.

Jennifer's Journey
Chapter 23

Jennifer is one of many I have spoken with, who after the death of a child, seeks a reversal. Another child cannot replace the one who was lost, but can help mend the pain and encourage the healing process. Here is Jennifer's story.

My journey starts back in 1993. I married the father of my oldest son, Brandon. I married because my mother was ill, and I wanted her to be at my wedding. Back then, I don't think it would have mattered who it was at the time, I would have said yes. My mom passed away in April 1994. Three weeks later, I found out I was pregnant with son number two. He was born December 1994, and I named him Tyler. Being a new mom again was the happiest I had been in a long time. My then husband was very abusive both physically and emotionally. He was also an alcoholic, though he would never admit it. My youngest son Tyler died of SIDS. Unfortunately, after he was born, I had my tubes tied. Now I was here with one son and quite simply knew that wasn't enough. I loved being a mom more than anything. My boys were, and always will be my life's meaning.

I had met a man while my marriage was reaching its end. I don't believe in love at first sight, but I knew when I met him, I wanted to be with him. He has always treated my son Brandon like his own, never wavering. We moved in together at the end of 1996 and married in June 2000, after five long years. We talked about having more children and the cost involved. We also discussed the affect it would have on Brandon. There was also my health to consider, as I have diabetes and am considered extremely high risk with my pregnancies.

I did some research online, and found Dr. Gary Berger and his clinic. I got the video and watched that. We discussed it with Keith's parents and my dad. I wanted to give my husband a child more than anything. This man is incredible, and I knew he would make a great daddy because of the way he was with my son. My son calls him daddy now, and I don't think anyone could love him more. He has said many times that he doesn't care whose DNA Brandon has, he is his son. They really are so much alike that most people don't know otherwise.

Keith's mom and dad, knowing what this meant to us and especially their son, gave us the money for the surgery. We had saved some up, but not enough. I called Dr. Berger's office and talked to them. They were a wealth of knowledge and full of compassion. They treated us like we were their only patient. Dr. Berger was so professional and caring. Travel there and cost of the surgery was very reasonable.

I obtained my chart and operative report from my tubal ligation doctor in Nashville. After receiving the report, Dr. Berger's office called stating they could do the surgery. We went for surgery on May 14, 2001. I was scared, but calm and excited all at the same time. I wondered would it work, would I be okay, and how long would it take? Well, my surgery took about an hour and a half, and I was pregnant by July 31, 2001. I was elated and excited to give Keith, the love of my life, the one thing I knew no one else could or had ever given him before. Dakota Keith Parton was born March 15, 2002. Then came another surprise. I found out I was pregnant again on Mother's Day. Noah Evan Parton was born December 15, 2003.

All of my children are handsome and beautiful, and of course, I was right, Keith is an awesome daddy. He loves being a daddy. He jokes, "If we could just get them to quit eating, I could be home full time, too." I have been a stay at home mom for four years, and I love it. Each day is filled with joy and hope. I learn more from my boys than anywhere else. Their innocence, their questions, and unconditional love makes me realize everyday I made the right choice.

Both babies were preemies. I was very sick and wasn't without pain. Dakota weighed only 4lbs, 14oz., and Noah, 4lbs., 7oz. They were only in the NICU for two weeks. We weren't sure if either I, or Noah, were going to make it at the end, but we did, and both boys are now huge, very intelligent, and have no lasting problems. The few they had early on had nothing to do with the reversal, but with my diabetes.

I believe Dr. Berger was put here for a reason, to help give us our own little angels. He is not God, but I believe God does lead him in his surgery and in his life. I feel like I am the luckiest woman, the happiest mom, and the most loved wife in the world.

Maura's Journey
Chapter 24

This story reminded me just how wonderful our God really is! He can take all the bad in our lives and bring good into it. Just more proof that we are never alone. God is always there to pull us out of the muck and mire, and always has an open door.

At the age of sixteen, I became a statistic and discovered that I was going to give birth to a baby in April 1990. Coming from a large Irish Catholic family, this was not a good thing. It was decided for me that the baby would be given up for adoption. After giving birth to a beautiful, healthy baby girl, I did just that.

Fast forward to January 1996. In a destructive, demeaning relationship, my then significant other and I, had convinced many doctors that I did not want any more children, that the adoption process had traumatized me beyond the pale, which was partly true. So at age 23, I had a tubal ligation. More aptly, I had them cauterized in four places, ensuring the impossibility of future pregnancies, along with an abdomnioplasty, which was major reconstructive surgery on my abdomen to erase all traces of my pregnancy. Essentially, I removed one scar, stretch marks, and replaced it with another, an eight inch scar.

Fast forward again to 2000. Solo and happy, I met and fell in love with the most unbelievable man in the entire universe, who despite my barren state, fell as equally in love with me. After discovering I was unable to have children, he embarked upon a mission, unbeknownst to me, to find a doctor who would make me whole again. I never thought I would actually want to have another child. I had been brutally damaged by the surrender of my daughter. Still to this day, and for all days to come, it will be painful. Another child would not take away that pain, but I realized I still had love to give to another part of me. I wanted to experience the true joy of pregnancy as it was meant to be. I had found someone who loved and valued me, despite my thoughts of me being damaged goods.

After having gone through a painful birth in 1990, and a massive reconstructive plastic surgery in 1996, I was hesitant about going under the knife yet again, despite the potential outcome. My then boyfriend, now husband, had sent for and gave to me an information packet from the Chapel Hill Tubal Reversal Center complete with a VHS tape showing a complete procedure from beginning to end. It also contained all background on Dr. Berger with countless testimonies, along with a success rate. Despite all this, I was doubtful. I lived in Boston and had access to a virtual, medical Mecca. Why would I take a chance with a total stranger, a doctor in whom I had to place my complete trust in without ever having met him? I retrieved my medical history and forwarded it to Dr. Berger. I had to wait and see if I even qualified for the surgery. It felt like the longest anticipated answer I can remember. What if my tubes had been so badly cauterized there was nothing left to fix? Would I die alone without ever having more children? Awful feelings, lonely feelings, sad, angry, indignant feelings swirled around me. I felt I was going crazy while I awaited the verdict from Dr. Berger. Why had I done this to my body? What was I thinking? Would Bob still want to be with someone who could never have children? Difficult and trying was the time that passed while I waited. As fate would have it, Dr. Berger found that I would be a good candidate for the surgery, so we arranged a date for the procedure.

Aside from the emotional commitment obstacle, the distance was a giant obstacle. I hate to fly and need medication before I even think about getting on a plane. My mother was to accompany me to the surgery. She was already on vacation in North Carolina, so she was going to meet me there. Not only could I not take medication 48 hours prior to surgery, I had to fly alone. Nearly two hours of self-doubt, recrimination, and a panic attack later, I arrived in North Carolina. My mother and I considered driving, but we determined that my well-being on the ride home would not allow for it. Another obstacle was the financial aspect. I had quit my job, and I returned to school full-time to get my undergraduate degree. I had just graduated, was engaged, and was not in a firm financial spot. As a marriage gift, not a wedding gift, my mother paid for everything-surgery, flight, and hotel included. It proved to be a worthy investment.

I was so nervous about surgery. I felt alone all over again. Sitting in a hospital gown in a pre-op room felt all too familiar. I returned to feelings of self-loathing. Why had I brought myself to this again? Why had I been so stupid in the past? What if it doesn't work?

Then, I saw Dr. Berger. He instantly made me feel so much better with his calm demeanor and reassuring way. Every nurse was steadfast in their kindness as well. After the surgery, all I wanted to do was sleep. The nurse brought us back to the hotel, medicated me, tucked me in, and off I drifted. She came back to check on me, and within 48 hours, give or take, I was preparing to return to Boston with a positive outlook from Dr. Berger. That was June 2001.

In April 2002, Bob and I were married. Again, I was plagued with the little voice in the back of my head. What if it didn't work? I had to relax and trust that as God had brought me to it, he would therefore bring me through it. We decided that the first year of marriage was going to be the year for us. We traveled to Maui and Kauai on our honeymoon. We traveled to the Bahamas, Cabo San Lucas, and finally to Nantucket on our one year anniversary. Prior to that trip, I went to see my doctor to tell her that we were going to start trying to get pregnant, two years post tubal reversal. She recommended an HSG, a procedure which demonstrates if the tubes are clear or blocked by injecting a dye into the uterus, and viewing on screen the reaction of the dye. It reflected one tube blocked, but one tube was free and clear. Three weeks later, I was pregnant!

Our reaction was complete happiness and borderline giddiness. To this day, Bob says, "I knew it would happen. I had no doubts all along." I, on the other hand, had my doubts. After so much disappointment in my life, I was hard pressed to believe that I would be rewarded with a healthy pregnancy. But there it was on the HPT strip, two lines, not one. I took a second test just to make sure, and as if it knew I doubted it, the two lines were even darker the second time around. I instantly became the delicate flower in my husband's eyes, and he could not do enough for me. The youngest child of seven, I shared the news with everyone at different times, and the response was overwhelming love, laughing, crying, and total excitement. My husband was able to tell his grandmother the day before she passed away that he was going to be a father. She smiled a smile that only a mother can understand.

Fast forward through a painfully sick and lumbering 9 months and 6 days. January 14, 2004, Samuel Finbarre Rogers, all 9lbs., 1 oz. of him, came screaming into the world. I knew in my heart of hearts that he would mend my heart of the pain it had long felt. I couldn't believe how much I loved this little nugget of love, this baby boy who has become our pal, our doodlebug, our little monkey. His smiles are our salve. Our love for him is endless, boundless, and at times all consuming. We are blessed to have him in our lives and show him our love everyday.

Job 6:8

Oh, that I might have my request, that God would grant what I hope for

Robin's Journey
Chapter 25

I am sure we can all relate to Robin's story in some way. Most of us have had family and friends who did all they could to encourage us to have a tubal ligation. Although intentions may have been good, in reality, they helped lead us to make a decision to rip our fertility out of the hands of the Maker Himself, and miss out on the chance to receive more of his most precious gifts. But luckily, God gave us a way to place our fertility back into his hands, where it belongs, and forgive us.

I had a tubal ligation after my third child. I was 23 years old. At the time, I really did not want to have the ligation done, but due to pressure from family members, I made the decision to go through with it. I complied because I was convinced that my family was complete. Three years later, my husband and I were divorced.

I remarried in 2001. My husband and I have always dreamed of having a baby together. I had my three sons, and he had his son, but we did not have one that we could call ours together. We talked about it for several years. We figured even if we ever could afford it, it would probably not be very successful. I had been told by many that reversing my tubal ligation would be next to impossible. My husband, Frank, on a venture to prove this wrong, got online one day and found Dr. Berger's website. He sent off for his video detailing the tubal reversal procedure. He then continued to look for other doctors that did the same surgery, but could not find any that he felt were as affordable, or as qualified as Dr. Berger.

Frank worked on the road back then. He called me one day while working and told me to call Dr. Berger's office and set up an appointment. He was ready to just do it! I was nervous, but made the call. They had just had a cancellation and could get me in the following week. I gathered the necessary paperwork from my tubal ligation surgery, and I went for all the necessary blood work. We left for Chapel Hill on a Wednesday, knowing we were about to change our lives forever.

On October 21, 2004, I had my tubal reversal. After the surgery, I was left with 4.5 cm of tube on my right side and 5 cm of tube on my left side. I thought these lengths were okay, but I was not very optimistic that I would ever get pregnant.

Someone had given me a copy of TCOYF. I read this book cover to cover. I then started taking my temperature each morning, checking cervical fluid, and placing it on my chart each day. I did everything the book suggested and then some. My night stand looked like a science project! I was taking Robitussin and baby aspirin. After trying to conceive for seven months we still were not pregnant, and I was quite depressed. The next month, I doubled my water intake to increase cervical fluid which made about a fifty percent difference, and we baby danced on the right days. After eight months trying to conceive, we were finally pregnant. Unfortunately, the pregnancy was diagnosed a blighted ovum, and we lost that baby in July 2004.

I was crushed that the pregnancy was not viable, but at the same time happy, knowing that the surgery was a success, and it was possible for me to become pregnant. We found out in October we were expecting again, three days before the anniversary of my reversal surgery date.

Roman Zane was born June 9, 2005, three weeks early. He weighed 6 lbs., 4 oz. Roman stayed seven days in the NICU before coming home to complete our family, which now numbered seven. Everyday, I look at my little baby and thank God for giving Dr. Berger the talent to put my tubes back together and for giving us this beautiful miracle. Frank and I could not be happier to have our Angelbutt baby!

Jeremiah 1:5

Before I formed you in the womb I knew you, before you were born I set you apart...

Liz's Journey
Chapter 26

Time and again, we hear of the high costs and long recovery time when having a tubal reversal. It just isn't so. I am hoping with stories like Liz's, that others will learn that they have more options, and not to give up when told a reversal is impossible, or a long, grueling recovery process. With God on your side, anything is possible. Here is Liz's story.

Let me take you back just 23 years. I have two boys from a previous marriage, who are now 21 and 23 years old. Being a single mom for several years and the struggles we went through, helped me to make the decision in 1990, to have a tubal ligation. At that time in my life, I felt that was the best decision for me. This brings me to my life now.

My husband Roy and I met eleven years ago and have been married for eight of those years. He had never been married, nor had any children of his own when we decided to get married. At that point and time in his life, he was content with that. His feelings changed several years later, which led us to make a very important decision, to have our baby, or move on.

Before we found Chapel Hill, we visited several places locally, only to be told that the surgery was going to be as extreme as open-heart surgery.

Recovery time, we were told, would be 6-8 weeks, and the cost would be over $10,000. This is the information we kept finding everywhere, so we started to lose hope. I wanted to have a baby by the time I turned 40, which wasn't too far off. I researched the internet and found Dr. Berger in Chapel Hill, North Carolina. We were never so thrilled to find that not only was it a quick recovery, but the success rate was great and the surgery very affordable. Having said that, I would like to thank my husband's Grandma, Louise, for making this dream come true for us by giving us the money we needed. As soon as we had everything prepared, we called Dr. Berger's office and made an appointment for the earliest day possible. Dr. Berger's staff was able to get us in the following month.

We both took a week off work and drove from Ohio to Chapel Hill. We had an appointment to visit the facility the day we arrived. I must say, Dr. Berger and his staff were wonderful to us. They all made us feel at home, as though we had known each other for years. My surgery was the next day, July 30, 2003. I was up and walking around just a few hours after surgery and was able to leave the following morning. There was some pain associated with the surgery. I don't want to come across as if there were none, but there was not as much as what you would think. The incision was small, maybe 3-4 inches in length, but it is worth it ladies! My results after surgery were 5 cm on the left tube and 7 cm on the right tube.

My husband and I gave it a month for recovery before we started trying to conceive. I found out I was pregnant in October 2003, but had a miscarriage, or ectopic, on November 22, 2003. The hospital was unsure as to whether it was ectopic or not. We scheduled a follow-up visit for an HSG to see if I had any damage or blocking.

The HSG was done in January 2004. It was at that time I found out my right tube was blocked. I only had my left to work with, but we didn't give up, we kept on trying. My concerns were future ectopic pregnancies. I didn't know how many times I could mentally go through the pain of losing my baby, but I tried not to let it discourage me. I had a goal to accomplish, and that was to bring a beautiful baby into this world, and I was determined to do so.

We were very lucky, because a month after my HSG, we found out I was pregnant again. We were very nervous this time because we lost the first baby. We kept our fingers crossed. I was monitored by my OBGYN on my HCG levels until they reached a high enough level to confirm a viable pregnancy.

I was closely watched throughout my pregnancy. I was considered high risk due to my age, but was taken off of high risk status after my fourth month. The pregnancy was going great! We had a 3D ultrasound done when I was 23 weeks pregnant so we could determine the sex. It was at this time we learned we were going to have a girl.

Lacy Janee was born November 2, 2004, at 7:05 p.m. She weighed 8lbs., 13oz. and was 21 inches long. She is our princess, our dream, our life! Don't ever give up, dreams come true!

Melanie's Journey
Chapter 27

Melanie is one of my tr sisters I have known since first seeking a reversal. She belonged to the first reversal group I joined on my search for support groups. Melanie and I shared due dates, my first baby, her second. We also shared delivery dates, just hours apart. She is one of a growing number of women going on to have several reversal blessings. Here is Melanie's story.

My tubal reversal journey began in December 1999. My husband introduced me to the internet. What a blessing that was! I think tubal reversal was the first thing I looked up. Ever since I had my tubal ligation back in 1991, months following the birth of my second child, I knew I had made a terrible mistake. All I wanted was to have things back the way they were. I asked around about having my ligation reversed, but all I ever got was negative responses. People told me it was too expensive, it couldn't be done, and even if I found a doctor that could perform the surgery, the chances of getting pregnant were very slim. So I never pursued the subject again, until December 1999. I dreamed of having more, never thinking it would ever come true.

Then, I found Dr. Berger's website. I soaked up all the information I could. I searched for other doctors, too, but always returned to Dr. Berger. I just felt the Lord was guiding me in his direction. I must have read his website 100 times over the next two months. Finally, in February 2000, I called to schedule an appointment. I couldn't believe this was really going to be happening. In a few months, I was going to be a whole woman again. It seemed like a dream. Every day I woke up counting the days down until my surgery. In the meantime, I obtained a copy of my pathology report, called my insurance company, checked on flights, and dreamed about the future. Dr. Berger sent me a VHS copy of a tubal reversal procedure he had performed. I had seen it on TLC and was very impressed, but anxious to watch it again.

Before I knew it, May was here, and my husband and I were on a flight to North Carolina. We met Dr. Berger the day before the surgery. My ligation reports were too vague and did not state what type of ligation I had, or if there was enough tube to repair. If Dr. Berger found that there was enough, he would proceed, if not, that would be the end of our journey. Needless to say, I was a nervous wreck. The nurses were all so nice. They made me feel comfortable and relaxed. The last thing I remember was the gas mask over my face and counting backward. I awoke from surgery to find that I was a whole woman again. My tubes were back together! I ended up with 5.5 cm of tube left on one side and 6.5 cm of tube left on the other. I was happy as could be and couldn't wait to get home. We stayed at the hotel for two nights. Dr. Berger came by each day to check on me and my progress. I was doing great, feeling great, and ready to take the flight home on Monday. After arriving home, I had to take it easy and rest a lot. Sitting down, or leaning over, was probably the hardest, but I knew it would all be worth it. Within two weeks, the swelling and tenderness was subsiding. After four weeks, I felt like myself again. My husband and I were anxious to conceive right away. We waited the first cycle and decided to start trying the next. I was very fortunate and got pregnant right away. My first reversal baby was born in March 2001. We got pregnant again four months later, but I miscarried before I was six weeks. I took it harder than I thought I would and put trying to conceive on hold for quite some time. We once again began trying to conceive in early 2002. After months of trying, we finally conceived. I gave birth to my second reversal baby in May 2003. My husband and I figured we better start early on our next baby, so we didn't waste any time. Our third reversal baby was born in August 2004.

Having three more children in our family is a feeling I cannot describe. At times, it seems so unbelievable, yet here they are. Sometimes I just look at them and can't believe they are mine. It is hard not to think of what once was. In my mind, I knew tubal ligation meant not having anymore children. I knew it, and I did it anyway. I really messed up. I thought I could handle the side effects from the tubal ligation. Having to live with the fact that I could no longer have children hit me harder and harder each passing year. I blamed myself for what I had done to my own body. Having to live with my own guilt was probably the hardest. I dealt with it the best I could and tried to move on. I was sure the yearning for more children would eventually go away. I am just thankful things worked out for the better. Having the tubal reversal has not only brought me peace of mind, but it has helped heal a part of my heart.

I am forever grateful to Dr. Berger and his staff. I thank God everyday for giving us people like Dr. Berger, and filling him with the knowledge and compassion to perform the work that he does. Chapel Hill Tubal Reversal Center has made my dreams come true. I will never forget that.

Micaela's Journey
Chapter 28

After a successful reversal surgery, Micaela and her husband discovered another obstacle in their way, her husband had his own fertility issues to work with. But, all in all, when it's the will of God, there will be a way. Here is Micaela's story.

I got my tubal ligation in May 1992, after my fourth child and a divorce from their father. My second husband, Max, who was also previously married, had no biological children of his own. He knew I could never have children, but accepted that and married me anyway.

About six years into our marriage, while on the internet, a pop up about tubal reversals came up. I went to the website and there was Dr. Berger. I was skeptical at first, not thinking this could be possible. Boy, was I ever wrong! I spoke to my husband about this new information and he was excited. I had a vacation coming up at work, so I called Dr. Berger's office, got all the paperwork together, and booked a flight to Chapel Hill after being told I would be a good candidate for a reversal. I flew in on Thursday for my consultation and had surgery on Friday. We found out one more problem, though. It turned out my husband's sperm count was low. We went back home to Florida wondering what we were going to do now. Dr. Berger called to see how we were doing and how my husband was doing. He then gave us the great news that there was help for my husband's problem. Dr. Berger called our primary care doctor, and he gave orders of what needed to be done. My husband had surgery as well. The urologist gave us about seven months to find out if the surgery would be successful.

My husband's surgery was March 12, 2002. March 26, 2002, I began to feel really sick. I went to my OBGYN in April, for my yearly exam, where my doctor gave me the news that I had "a loaf of bread" in the oven. I did not understand at that point what he meant. He then had some blood work done to confirm the pregnancy. When the test came back positive, all I could do was cry and scream with joy.

My husband came home that night and asked what was for dinner. He hadn't realized I had been crying when I handed him his dinner. He looked at me and asked what in the world was going on, and why did I hand him a Happy Meal for dinner? I told him to look inside the box, and there I placed the proof we had so long waited for.

About six months into my pregnancy, I ran into some complications. I was admitted for two days to prevent labor, then was sent home. My baby was due January 3, 2003, but while Christmas shopping on December 23rd, my water broke. The baby was stuck under my rib cage, so a c-section was done to ensure a safe delivery. There she was, Cecilya SJ Alvarado, all 6 lbs., 11 oz., and 21 inches of her. That was the greatest feeling of joy I ever experienced in life. She is now almost three years old. I owe a big thanks to Dr. Berger, and his staff. I have referred eleven people to Dr. Berger since my surgery, and all eleven have been successful as well.

Mark 11:24

Therefore I tell you, whatever you ask for in prayer, believe that you have received it, and it will be yours.

Holly's Journey
Chapter 29

Holly's story is a tear-jerker. After losing her middle son to Leukemia, she was desperate for another child. When adoption proved to be more than they could afford, they turned to tubal reversal surgery and were blessed with another child to help mend the pain. Here is Holly's story.

My name is Holly Kindell. I was 33 years old when Dr. Berger performed my tubal reversal surgery. My tubes had been tied for ten years. I had my tubal ligation after the birth of my third son. I had reluctantly made the decision, knowing my husband didn't want any more children. I have always wanted more children. Anyway, I had the ligation surgey, and always regretted it.

My middle son, Adam, was diagnosed with Acute Lymphoblastic Leukemia in 1996. My husband, myself, and the other children were tested to see if any of our bone marrow matched Adams. We did not. I wished then that I could have another child to see if that one would match. Because none of us were a match, we began chemotherapy treatments, and were told that Adam had a great chance of beating the cancer because of the fact that he was only three, and it was only in his bone marrow. After two years of treatment, Adam relapsed in his spinal fluid. Ultimately, after three relapses, an unrelated bone marrow transplant, and eight years of treatment, we lost Adam on December 21, 2003.

We were completely devastated! I especially was lost. I felt like I had no purpose anymore. I had spent the last eight years of his life taking care of him. He hadn't been able to go to school a lot of the time, so were together a lot. I was so used to always having Adam with me. My other boys pretty much learned to take care of themselves. I pleaded with my husband, Doug, for another child. Doug agreed we should look into adoption, but it was way too expensive.

One day, while on the internet, I looked up tubal reversal and found Dr. Berger's website. I was very impressed with the price and the odds of a successful surgery. Doug and I agreed that it was the best way to go. I made the payment and set things into motion for that May. We flew in on a Thursday to meet Dr. Berger. I was very impressed with his compassion and concern. The hotel we stayed in was very nice. My husband had a great time exploring Chapel Hill. Saturday, May 7th was my surgery. Again, I was so impressed with Dr. Berger and his staff. They do everything possible to ensure the comfort of their patients, before, during, and after surgery. The nurses were great!

I flew home the next day with only minimal soreness. I was back to my old self within a couple of weeks. After only four months of trying to conceive, I was pregnant. We were elated! I was so afraid the pregnancy was tubal because of an increased risk, but that wasn't the case. I gave birth May 30th to a healthy 7 lb., 13 oz. baby boy, who we named Wyatt Adam. He was born a year and thirteen days from my surgery date. We are very thankful to God for leading us to Dr. Berger.

Hebrews 11:1

Now faith is being sure of what we hope for and certain of what we do not see.

Quick Testimonies
Chapter 30

My name is Teresa. I had my reversal surgery in December 2001, with Dr. Berger. I had my ligation after my third child in 1990. My ligation was "ringed." I remarried in 1999, and decided to try the reversal. I had the surgery in December and was pregnant in January. Unfortunately, I miscarried at nine weeks. I was pregnant two months later and gave birth to my son on March 20, 2003. After breastfeeding for a year, we decided to try again. I was 41 by now. I got pregnant right away, then had a miscarriage at 14 weeks. Again, I was pregnant within two months, and we had our last son July 14, 2005. I feel like I've been pregnant four years. I had quick success with the reversal despite my "advanced" age. I'm 43 now, and wondering if I should get my tubes ringed again to prevent another pregnancy! This should be an inspiration to other women who are wondering about fertility after reversal surgery. It can, and does work very well!

My name is Misty. I had my tubal ligation with Hulka Clips in 1999, after having my twins, but wasn't able to have a reversal until June 17, 2003. We had to save up the money and wanted to do plenty of research to find the best doctor for me, which was Dr. Berger. It was a hard time for me because I wanted to share a child so much with the man I loved more than anything. I was thrilled when I was finally able to make the appointment. After surgery, I was back to myself in about one week. I had 6 cm left on each side. I conceived the next cycle, about three weeks later. My pregnancy was great with no problems whatsoever. I delivered Brandon Matthew Bowling on April 8, 2004, at 12:32 p.m. He weighed 8 lbs., 7 oz., and was 20 ¾ inches long. He is such a blessing to our entire family.

My name is Ann. I am 36 years old, and my husband of fourteen years is 40. We both have grown children from previous marriages. I always wanted a child with my husband, but raising four children without the help of the other parents was expensive. We knew we could not afford the surgery, or the expense it would take to raise another child. As time went on, I heard more and more about reversal surgery. I went online to find more information out about this surgery. By 2003, we were able to afford the surgery and raise another child. I researched several reversal doctors, but Dr. Berger seemed the right choice for us. The cost was reasonable, the recovery time short, and it was close enough to drive from Baltimore to Chapel Hill. I thought this was too good to be true. Everything happened very quickly. I had surgery on Wednesday, September 24, 2003, and was back to work that Monday. I was pregnant three months later, and had my precious little miracle, Tony Jr., on September 26, 2004. He is our ray of sunshine everyday. If I had to do this over again, I would not change a thing. Good luck to all thinking about a reversal. I would recommend Dr. Berger to anyone.

My name is Dawn. I had my tubal ligation after my middle son was three years old, not thinking I would ever want another child. Well guess what, nine years later, I did. I did some research online and found Dr. Berger. Our journey began August 20, 2002. After surgery, my tube lengths were 4 cm and 6 cm. The following month we started trying to conceive. Sadly to say, for six months, no pregnancy. An HSG in February proved both tubes to be open. I took Clomid for months, with no success. In June, July, and August, we had an IUI, which failed all three times. After more testing and finding nothing wrong, I was very disappointed. My doctor told me the only thing he can do besides IVF was to put me on Metformin, which is a drug they use for gestational diabetes. He said some fertility doctors prescribe it for infertility with good results. It is also used for women with PCOS. We figured, why not give it a try? Ten days later, I was finally pregnant after thirteen months. I delivered a healthy 6 lb., 3 oz., and 21 inch long baby boy on May 30, 2004. I recently went back to my OBGYN and got put back on the medication. My doctor thinks I probably do have PCOS with a couple of the symptoms. It has been fifteen months since the birth of our son, and we are still working on reversal baby two.

John 16:21

A woman giving birth to a child has pain because her time has come; but when her baby is born she forgets the anguish because of her joy that a child is born into the world.

Learn the Lingo

Here are a list of some of the many abbreviations we TR sisters use when communicating online:

AF-Aunt Flo (meaning menstrual cycle or period)

BBT-Basal Body Temperature

BD-Baby Dance (the act of trying to conceive)

BETA-blood test for pregnancy, measures HCG levels

BFN-Big Fat Negative (this is bad)

BFP-Big Fat Positive (this is good)

CD-Cycle Day (menstrual cycle day)

CL-Coverline (on temperature chart)

CM-Cervical Mucus (same as fluid)

CF-Cervical Fluid (same as mucus)

DD-Dear Daughter

DH-Dear Husband or sometimes Darned Husband

DS-Dear Son

DPO-Days Past/Post Ovulation

EDD-Estimated/Expected Due Date

EPO-Evening Primrose Oil (cm helper)

EWCM-Egg-white Mucus (most fertile)

FMU-First Morning Urine

FSH-Follicle Stimulating Hormone

GnRH-Gonadotropin Releasing Hormone

HCG-Human Chorionic Gonadotropin

HPT-Home Pregnancy Test

HSG-Hysterosalpinogram

LAP-Laparoscopy

LH-Leutenizing Hormone (detected by OPK)

LMP-Last Menstrual Period

LOL-Laughing Out Loud

LP-Luteal Phase (Days between O and AF)

M/C-Miscarriage

O-Ovulation

OPK-Ovulation Predictor Kit (detects LH surge)

PCOS-Polycystic Ovarian Syndrome

PCT-Post Coital Test

PG-Pregnant!

POAS-Potty On A Stick (PG test)

PMS-Pre-Menstrual Syndrome

PROG-Progesterone

RE-Reproductive Endocrinologist

RX-Prescription

ROBI-Robitussin (helps with CM)

SA-Sperm Analysis

SAHM-Stay At Home Mom

TCOYF-Book you gotta have!

TTC-Trying To Conceive

US-Ultrasound

TL-Tubal Ligation (big no-no)

TR-Tubal Reversal (big yes)

VBAC-Vaginal Birth After C-Section

2WW-Two Week Wait (O to hopefully PG)

Angels Helping Others

I ran across this wonderful group of women a short time ago. Angels Helping Others is a group of women on a mission to help fund tubal reversals for those who otherwise would not financially be able. In the short time I have been with these ladies, I have seen mountains moved. God's hand is definitely in this ministry.

I, speaking for myself, do believe that tubal ligation is wrong. Our fertility belongs in the hands of our Creator, God. We cannot change the mistake we made in the past, but I do believe God will hold us accountable for what we decide to do once we realize our mistake.

I would like to ask you to check out their websites, and if God places it upon your heart to help support the efforts of Angels Helping Others, I would invite you to do so.

www.angelshelpingothers.com

Donations are greatly appreciated! You can also purchase items at www.cafepress.com/trfundstore as a way to show your support!

Luke 1:37

For nothing is impossible with God!